MW00325739

FAITH, HOPE AND CANCER

THE JOURNEY OF A CHILDHOOD CANCER SURVIVOR

CAROLYN KONCAL BREINICH

Copyright © 2018 Carolyn Koncal Breinich

All rights reserved. No part of this publication may be reproduced, distributed or transmitted in any form or by any means, including photocopying, recording, digital scanning, or other electronic or mechanical methods, without prior written permission of the publisher, except in the case of brief quotations embodied in critical reviews and certain other noncommercial uses permitted by copyright law. For permission requests, please contact the author at www.leukemiagirl.com

Published in 2020

Printed in the United States of America

ISBN: 978-1-7347804-9-9 (hardcover)

ISBN: 978-1-7347804-1-3 (softcover)

ISBN: 978-1-7347804-2-0 (ebook)

Library of Congress Control Number: 2020904144

Scripture references marked as ESV were taken from The ESV® Bible (The Holy Bible, English Standard Version®), copyright © 2001 by Crossway, a publishing ministry of Good News Publishers. Used by permission. All rights reserved.

Scripture references marked LTB were taken from The Living Bible copyright © 1971 by Tyndale House Foundation. Used by permission of Tyndale House Publishers Inc., Carol Stream, Illinois 60188. All rights reserved.

Cover Art by Michelle Shaw

Edited by Meredith Tennant and Judith Schwartz

CONTENTS

AUTHOR'S NOTE

This book is a memoir. It reflects the author's present recollections of experiences over time. Occasionally, dialogue consistent with the character or nature of the person speaking has been supplemented. All persons within are actual individuals; there are no composite characters. The names of some individuals have been changed to respect their privacy.

ACKNOWLEDGMENTS

I would like to thank first and foremost my husband, Lee. You believed in me enough to allow me to pursue my dreams and gave me the opportunity to write this book. To my parents—for always being there for me and supporting me every step of the way. To my doctors and nurses at Children's Hospital—thank you for saving my life. To all the patients I worked with over the years—I will never forget you. To my Fred Astaire family—you welcomed me with open arms and showed me how to live again. To Gena—for helping me face my fears and giving me the motivation and strength to finish this book.

PREFACE

I consider January 25, the day I was diagnosed with cancer, as my second birthday and my day to celebrate life and thank God for what He has given me. Some choose to celebrate the day they went into remission, and some don't celebrate at all. I celebrate my diagnosis day because if that day had never happened, I wouldn't be here sharing my story. I wrote my first "cancerversary" email in 2001, to celebrate my seventh year of being a childhood cancer survivor. I was about to turn twenty-one and I felt the need to go out into the world and share my good news. I wanted to celebrate life, God's plan for me, the mysterious ways in which He works, and most importantly remind others to celebrate their lives. Email and the internet were becoming more popular, and I had a way to share my good news with a wide range of people who had been with me throughout my journey. Every year since then, I have continued to write a cancerversary email on that day.

Over the years, the list of people who receive my email has grown, and many have encouraged me to write a book. I have always known sharing my story could provide hope or inspire others, but I never considered myself a writer. Until now. I am a firm believer that everything happens for a reason. This book is no exception.

In 2016, my husband gave me the greatest gift: the gift to quit my job and follow my dream. For the first two weeks after I quit my job, the words just flowed. In a short period of time, I had the first rough draft of this book written. Then it came to a screeching halt. I hadn't prepared myself for the emotions that came along with the memories. For a year, I wanted to work on the book but was too afraid to face the emotions again. Then I heard a former classmate had been diagnosed with breast cancer. I had to reach out to her. I knew the words in my book could offer her hope. Her diagnosis gave me the courage to open my book and start rereading some of the chapters. I was pleasantly surprised that even though the memories were there, the accompanying emotion had decreased. I was not only able to help her and her family, but I was able to move forward and finish writing my story.

My journey wasn't an easy one. I survived before the internet connected people and before organizations existed to help survivors. I want to show you how having faith in something greater and hope for a better future changed my life, and how it can and will get you through the hard times.

Life will always have its ups and downs, but it is how we respond to the highs and lows that shapes us into who we are. Those who read this book will laugh, cry, and be inspired. You will gain a perspective on what a child (or anyone) diagnosed with cancer goes through. You will see how hope and faith are important keys to survival. Even though my journey wasn't always easy, I would do it all over again, knowing I am here now, sharing it with you.

MIRACLES DO HAPPEN

*E*veryone has a defining moment in their life, a moment that changed the course of their life. I was thirteen when I first experienced that feeling and my life changed. Up until then, I lived what I considered a normal life. I grew up in the suburbs, the youngest of three, without a care in the world. I dreamt of becoming a veterinarian, getting married, having two children and many dogs. I was happy living the life my parents provided me. Nothing prepared me for the path my life was about to take.

November 1993. I was in the eighth grade at basketball practice. That night, I was kneed in the back while guarding a teammate. I immediately felt a sharp pain in my lower back and asked my coach if I could get some water and sit down. I walked to the drinking fountain and then sat on the bleachers waiting for practice to be over. When my mom picked me up, I told her what happened and about the pain. My parents assumed I had just pulled a muscle. I ended up staying home from school the next day because the pain was still there. I just couldn't get comfortable.

A week later, my parents took me to see our family doctor to determine if there was internal damage since I was not getting better and continued to feel a sharp pain in my back. He took x-rays, but nothing showed up, so rest, heat, and aspirin were recommended.

For the next month, I dealt with the pain the best way I could. I didn't swallow pills, so my parents crushed over-the-counter pain medication and I mixed it with a spoonful of sugar. (Mary Poppins was wrong: a spoonful of sugar does not make the medicine go down.) Crushed medicine tastes horrible, but because it was the same color as sugar, I only took a quarter of the crushed medication with the sugar. I didn't tell anyone what I was doing. I didn't want my parents to worry, so I pretended to feel better. I thought the pain was temporary and I could just live with it. Boy, was I wrong.

In December, I began sleeping in a recliner in our family room because I couldn't lie down. It hurt too much to lie flat on a bed. When I was home, I lived in that chair. It was the only place I had some comfort, although the pain was still present. One night I felt better and decided to try sleeping in my bed. Big mistake. The pain escalated and I couldn't sit up and get out of bed. Instead, I slowly rolled and then used the edge of the bed to stand. I knew something was wrong. I knew this wasn't normal, and I also knew no one could tell me why I was in so much pain.

After playing in one scrimmage basketball game, I realized I had to quit the team. I knew I wasn't going to be able to play—the pain was too severe. I had been playing basketball since the fourth grade; I didn't want to give it up. I didn't want the pain to win, but it did. I sat on my parents' bed, picked up the phone and called the coach. As we talked, I think he understood why I felt the need to quit, but I knew my teammates wouldn't.

Basketball was the first thing I had to give up. A couple weeks later, as I was helping my mom set up for Secret Santa (The Christmas activity she organized for kids to shop for their family during school), the pain in my back hurt so bad I was in tears and just wanted to go home. Since my mom was in charge, she couldn't leave to take me home, so I was stuck at school in unbearable pain and couldn't do anything about it. Good thing God had other plans. Mr. Tonti, one of our neighbors and a coach at the school, happened to come down to the gym where we were setting up. I believe God sent him there so he could take me home. He was there so I didn't have to sit in pain waiting for my mom to finish. I was heartbroken leaving and not being able to help with Secret Santa. It was a Christmas tradition and something I had been a part of since I was four years old. I didn't feel I had a choice; the pain was now controlling my life.

I continued going to school despite the constant pain. My school made accommodations for me, such as letting my books remain in the classroom, eliminating the need for me to carry them from class to class. At the time, my class had to carry all our books with us as we were not allowed to go to our lockers during the day. My mom had weighed my bookbag, and it weighed forty pounds. It was then I was given an extra set of books to keep at home, so I didn't need to carry anything home.

This was the beginning of feeling set apart from my classmates. They didn't understand why I received special treatment. They didn't understand how severe my back pain was. All they knew was what I told them: I had a sharp, stabbing pain that moved to different parts of my back. One minute it would be in my upper back, the next minute in my lower back or in the middle. Then, I over-heard a friend say, "Real pain doesn't move." It was at that moment I realized they thought I was faking. I couldn't understand why they thought this, and unfortunately, I had no way to prove the pain was real.

Even my siblings didn't believe the pain was real, or at least they didn't believe the pain was as intense as I claimed. Being the youngest, my sister and brother viewed me as the baby of the family, the one who would cry to get what I wanted. Over the course of the month, my brother, Steven, went on with his life. He was a junior in high school and had other things to worry about than his younger sister getting kneed in the back at basketball prac-tice and having back pain. Theresa was a freshman in college, lived two hours away and had no idea what I was experiencing. She came home from college to see me sleeping in a chair. I can only assume she thought my parents were babying me once again.

One day when the three of us were upstairs, they pushed me into the wall to see if the pain was real. I fell backwards hitting my back on the doorknob of the clothes chute. I cried because of the pain it caused, but more importantly, I cried because I had no way to prove to anyone what I was going through. I just wanted people to believe me.

I tried to act normal because I wanted to feel normal. I wanted to feel included. What my family and friends didn't know was that I was hiding how bad it actually hurt. It hurt to laugh, sneeze, move quickly, sit on the bus, sit in the car, and sleep in a bed. Everything I did caused me pain; pain I wouldn't wish on my worst enemy. I never knew where the pain would be, and I never knew how intense it was going to be. The pain could go from a deep, aching pain to a sharp, stabbing pain at any minute. I took one day at a time and did the best I could.

I had countless x-rays, none of which showed anything wrong. Some suspected I had inherited a bad back, since my dad and other relatives had bad backs. My parents just figured it was an undetected slipped disk or growing pains. I knew what I was going through wasn't growing pains.

Come Christmas, all I wanted was a day without pain. Our family tradition was to wake up Christmas morning, open presents, eat cookies, and drive two hours to see our grandparents. I loved Christmas. It was and continues to be my favorite time of the year, but I was not looking forward to this particular Christmas. It hurt to be in a car for just ten minutes, let alone two hours. The seats were uncomfortable and each time the car went over a bump, I felt a sharp, stabbing pain in my back. The only thing I prayed for was a day without pain. I didn't care what Santa brought me; I was just tired of hurting.

Christmas morning I got my first miracle: I woke up without pain. For the first time in two months, I could move freely. I could sit on the ground. I could twist and turn. I thanked God for the greatest gift I could have been given. I opened my presents with my family, ate cookies, and survived the two-hour drive to see my grandparents without pain. Christmas morning, I learned miracles do happen.

THE C WORD

*S*adly, the pain didn't stay away for long. On New Year's Eve I was at my best friend Sam's house celebrating. We spent the day together, and I did my best to have a good time even though I was miserable. The intensity of the pain started to become more consistent. I wondered why my pain had returned, if I would ever know the cause, and if something was seriously wrong with me. I was afraid the sharp, stabbing pain was here to stay. I did my best to hide how I felt. I did my best to cope. I wanted to be normal. I wanted to have fun with my best friend. I sat there shifting my weight while we played games, watched TV, and took pictures of each other. No matter what I did, I couldn't find a comfortable position.

Just before midnight, the pain got so unbearable I called my parents to come get me because I knew I wouldn't be able to sleep on the floor at Sam's house. I'm sure he was mad at me for leaving, but I just couldn't stay. I felt horrible for letting him down. As much as I did not want it to, the pain ruled my life. Looking at the picture he took of me that day, so pale and thin, I wondered how no one realized I was sick.

For the next couple of weeks, the pain continued to control my life, people continued to have their doubts, and I just lived with it. Then on January 12, everything changed again. At the end of math class, I reached under my desk to get something out of my book bag and couldn't get up again. I was stuck hunched over. I tried sitting up, but I couldn't. I couldn't straighten my back. It was the most intense and excruciating pain I had felt. It felt as if someone had stuck a screwdriver in my spine, preventing me from straightening it. I was terrified. I looked to my friends for help, but I didn't see looks of sympathy or empathy on their faces; instead I saw laughter. I couldn't understand why they thought it was so funny. They all left for lunch, leaving me alone with the teacher.

The school nurse and my mom, who was the music teacher at my school, were called to the classroom. My mom called Theresa, who was home from college, to come pick me up. By the time she got to school, the pain had subsided enough, and I was able to sit up and walk out to the car. I know my friends saw me walking, which I thought confirmed their belief that I was faking, but for me, not being able to sit up was the scariest moment of my life, and my friends had done nothing to help. I became even more alienated from them.

The following day, another set of x-rays showed nothing wrong. Since this doctor couldn't tell us what was causing my pain and more specifically, what prevented me from straightening my back, my parents decided to take me to an orthopedic surgeon they knew and trusted. They called his office to set up an appointment, but he was out of town for the next two weeks. My parents asked if I could cope for two more weeks; I said yes, and they scheduled an appointment. I continued to live with the pain because I felt I didn't have a choice. We had a couple of snow days where I was able to stay home and rest, but finding a comfortable position was getting harder and harder. I spent the majority of my time in our recliner, sleeping or watching TV because I didn't have the energy, desire, or ability to do much else.

As time went on, the pain worsened and it no longer moved; instead, my entire back was in constant pain. I returned to school, with more special accommodations. I could skip gym class first period. I didn't want to go to school, I didn't want to be around my friends, and I didn't want to sit on the hard classroom chairs. The pain was so constant and so intense that it took over my life. I couldn't do anything anymore. I just wanted to find out what was wrong with me.

Monday, January 24, 1994, started out like every other day. My dad went to work, my brother drove my mom to her school and then he drove to his high school, and I was home with our dog. Around 9:00 a.m., I got up and walked to the bathroom to get ready for school. When I put my skirt on, the "screwdriver-in- my-back" feeling returned and again I couldn't straighten my back to stand. I was terrified, more terrified than the previous time because I was alone. No one was around to help me. I quickly sat, hunched over on the edge of the bathroom counter to ease the pain. I sat there with tears rolling down my cheeks because I was alone, the telephone was in the family room, and I was in excruciating pain.

After a couple of minutes, even though I was in the worst pain of my life, I forced myself to carefully walk back to the recliner knowing I had to call my dad. The phone was on the floor next to the chair. I sat there struggling to figure out how to get the phone off the floor. A simple task turned into an incredible obstacle when I couldn't lean over, bend, or move my upper back without being in excruciating pain. I carefully used my toes to pick up the phone by the antenna. I called my dad, crying in pain.

Within minutes he was home. A year earlier, he had been transferred to an office five minutes from our house. I think of this as another miracle. He walked in the door, told me he had had enough, and said, "We're going to the emergency room." He picked me up and carried me to the car. For the next five or six hours we sat in the emergency room at the local hospital. Upon check-in, the nurse took my temperature in my ear, which I thought was cool since I didn't know you could do that. I had blood work taken and they asked me to pee in a cup. The nurse was impressed that I balanced the urine cup on the toilet paper holder. Strange how I remember that.

As we waited, I begged Dad to call Mom. I love my dad, but he isn't the comforting type. He isn't one to sit and hold your hand; that's what my mom is for. My dad is the provider, the supervisor, the supporter. These are qualities I have since learned to appreciate and love. We didn't have cell phones back then, so Dad left a message on our answering machine at home for Mom. When she and Steven got home from school, they heard the message and Mom came to the hospital. By that time, I had been there for hours. She walked into the room and immediately commented on how my skin color matched the gray color of the walls and asked my dad when did my color get so ashen.

A few hours later, a doctor came to tell my parents, "You have a very sick daughter. It looks like she could either have aplastic anemia or leukemia. She could stay here, but I recommend getting her to Children's Hospital as soon as possible." I didn't comprehend what the doctor said; I just knew I was sick with something very bad. That moment our lives changed. Mom and Dad made the decision to take me to Children's Hospital. As much as Mom wanted to stay with me in the ER, she knew she needed to get home to start packing things and make phone calls about missing work the next day. Dad and I stayed to get the paperwork taken care of.

When Dad and I finally arrived home, Steven was just standing in the kitchen with a look of disbelief watching everything happen. I could tell he was worried, but at this point there was nothing he could do. Mom told Steven they were taking me to the hospital, and they would leave him a car to drive to school the next morning. Mom packed an overnight bag and I grabbed my stuffed dog Katie and toucan Puff-a-Lump. I said goodbye to Steven and to my dog Misty and we drove to the Children's Hospital emergency room. We were there a couple more hours until we finally got a room sometime after midnight. Sitting in the hospital bed was the first time I had a chance to really process and comprehend what was happening. The past few hours had been a blur. We were all in survival mode and did what we needed to get me to the hospital as quickly as possible, not knowing how sick I really was.

I sat in the bed looking around, I was in room 504 and there was a raccoon painting on the white walls. My bed was next to the window. I was in a shared room and a curtain divided the room in half. I was grateful no one was in the other bed as I didn't want to share my room with anyone. There was a TV, but no clock, which I thought was odd. There was a pullout chair Mom could use as a bed. After my nurse helped us get settled, Dad went home, and it was just Mom and me and a new stuffed bear I named Sickie. Sickie was a gift from the admissions department. Mom picked it out for me since she knew I loved stuffed animals. Sickie got her name because I was too sick to think of one. Mom and I were exhausted, both physically and emotionally. We quickly fell asleep.

The next morning I woke up to more blood tests. We went to the treatment room down the hall where I was to have my first lumbar puncture (spinal tap) and bone marrow biopsy. I laid on the table holding my stuffed dog and was given anesthesia to put me to sleep. When I woke up, I was told the doctor had to climb onto the treatment table to get the leverage he needed to get my bone marrow because it was too thick to flow through the syringe. I didn't know what that meant, but I was guessing it wasn't normal. I was also told that during the procedure I purred like a kitten while a nurse comforted me by rubbing my leg. It was then I learned that you can do strange things when given local anesthesia.

From there, it was a waiting game. I waited for nurses to bring me pain medication and I waited to find out what was wrong with me. Luckily, I didn't have to wait long. My doctor came in and delivered the news: acute lymphocyctic leukemia. Further tests revealed I had more specifically pre-pre-B cell cALLa positive acute lymphocyctic leukemia. Cancer. I had cancer!

I immediately felt a sense of relief. It didn't matter I had cancer. All that mattered was that I had proof my pain was real and they knew what was causing it. I didn't understand how serious cancer was, because I had never known anyone who had cancer. My only understanding of cancer was a story we had read in English class a few months earlier about a girl who had leukemia, had treatment, and survived. To me cancer was a good thing, because if it caused my pain, it also meant my pain would be gone once I started treatment.

My doctor went on to tell us the leukemia was causing

my pain, and I had very little healthy bone marrow. My bone marrow was 99 percent leukemia cells and I was lucky because there is only a small window of time in which to diagnose this type of leukemia. If I had had blood work done earlier during previous doctor visits, it would not have shown leukemia cells, and they would not have had any reason to retake my blood in the emergency room. He also said if I had not been diagnosed when I was, I likely would have gone into a coma and died within three days, more or less. I never would have seen my fourteenth birthday, which I celebrated five days later with my friends. A hospital isn't the best place to have a party, but it's better than not having a birthday at all.

The girl in the story we read lost her hair, so my first question to the doctor was "Am I going to lose my hair?" (I never liked my hair: It was too thin, and I never could do anything with it), followed by "I'm not going to have to do a science fair project this year." I was supposed to be working on my hypothesis and experiments but had been in too much pain to start, so I was behind. Cancer would get me out of completing the project.

My parents had many questions, although I only remember one. They asked if being diagnosed with leukemia was better or worse than having anemia, because those were the two options they had been given at the other hospital. My mom was surprised when my doctor said leukemia was the better of the two. My doctor explained that leukemia is treatable and curable whereas anemia is not. Anemia would have been a lifelong diagnosis. My dad asked more questions than my mom. Like me, she didn't comprehend the seriousness of what was happening. She stayed with me in the hospital while Dad went home to call the family. He called Theresa first, followed by grandparents, aunts, and uncles. I can only imagine what those phone calls were like. Mom called her principal to inform her that she would not be able to teach for the next couple of weeks, and that I would not be returning to school.

My diagnosis changed my whole life. I was bombarded with so many new experiences at once. I had never been in a hospital before, I had never taken so many pills before, and most of all, I had never been that scared before. I wasn't scared of the leukemia but of all the new things going on around me. All the new people, new concepts, and most of all the new lifestyle. In a matter of hours, the way I thought about life changed. I felt I had lost all control of my body. The control had been placed in the hands of my doctors, and in turn, I counted on them to get me better.

Cancer is a terrible thing, but when you're diagnosed with it, you can't focus on the idea it might kill you. You need to remain as positive as you can so you can get through the treatment.

From the beginning, I saw the positives in my diagnosis. I saw the positives because of my Catholic upbringing and because I finally had validation my pain was real. The doctors knew what was causing it and could do something to get rid of it. Shortly after my diagnosis, Mom said she believed I was chosen by God from all the students in my class to be able to handle this, especially since most would not have wanted to lose their hair. It was easy to be positive because I didn't know anything else.

I had been raised with the understanding of the power of prayer and trusted everything would work out in the end. Prayer was part of our daily routine; we prayed in school, before dinner, and when I went to bed. If I heard a siren, I prayed for those involved; if I saw a beautiful sunset, I thanked God for my eyes. Prayer came naturally to me. Faith was talked about in my family. I witnessed my grandparents reading their book of prayers every night and their faith in knowing God would take care of everything. Having cancer was no different. I prayed that God would take care of me. I didn't know how He would, I just knew He would. Prayer became one of my coping mechanisms.

Prior to being diagnosed, the only bad thing I had ever witnessed was Brian, a seminarian and a close family friend, deal with a life-changing event a year earlier. Even though the world appeared to be out to get him, he remained positive and faithful. Brian constantly said he knew God was with him. He didn't understand what God was doing, but he knew there was a reason he had to go through such a hardship. He had totally surrendered to God, trusting He was going to take care of everything. Brian was the second person to visit me in the hospital. He quickly said that he went through what he did so I could witness his faithfulness to God. Brian also told me that I would be a witness of God's love to others. He gave my cancer a purpose. He gave me hope that one day I would know the reason I was diagnosed. Throughout his whole ordeal and now my cancer diagnosis, he remained positive. Mom fed off his positivity and I fed off hers. If Brian could face such a life-changing event with such faith and determination, so could I.

I quickly accepted the fact I had cancer. I knew there wasn't anything I could do but put my faith in God, my doctors, and chemotherapy. I didn't go through the seven stages of grief, because I skipped right to the seventh stage —acceptance. One person who understood this was Father Ralko, the hospital chaplain. Right away he saw how God played a big part in my life, and he saw prayer was one of my coping mechanisms. He was also the only one to ask why my mom had a funeral planning book at my bedside. Apparently, the hospital staff assumed my mom thought I was dying and was getting ready to plan my funeral. While everyone else made assumptions about my mom, Father Ralko asked questions. Mom explained that her father was extremely sick and close to the end of his life. She was getting ready to help her mom prepare for his funeral. Luckily, my grandpa recovered and lived another year. We never did tell him how sick I was; all he knew was I was getting better.

Every day I looked forward to seeing Father Ralko. He brought me Communion, talked to me, and laughed with me. He understood me. We talked about death and how I wasn't afraid of it, we talked about life, we talked about everything. He also offered me the Sacrament of the Anointing of the Sick, which is a special blessing for health and comfort given to those who are sick or who have a life-threatening illness. Even though I had gone to Catholic school, I did not know much about this sacrament. After all, why would a kid need it? After receiving this sacrament, I felt a sense of peace and comfort knowing God was with me.

3

THE INITIAL HOSPITALIZATION

*T*here were a lot of procedures in the beginning, bone marrow biopsies, spinal taps, echocardiograms, EKGs, blood tests . . . all things to find out if the chemo was working, how far the leukemia had spread, and if my other organs were being affected. Most kids go to the treatment room for these procedures, but because of the pain I was in, they did many of these procedures in my room. This is an example of the great care at Children's Hospital.

Three days after my diagnosis, I had surgery to place a Broviac catheter (long-term central line) in my chest so the chemo could be given intravenously. When I woke up, I had a catheter with two small tubes (lumens) sticking out of my chest. The whole upper right part of my chest was bruised. I asked my mom what had happened, and she told me the surgeon was called to check on my Broviac in the recovery room because I wouldn't stop bleeding. At that time, he applied pressure to stop the bleeding, leaving a bruise the size of his hand on my chest.

It was great having a Broviac. Each lumen had a

removable cap and plastic clamp, and medications and blood products were injected through the caps into the catheter instead of an intravenous (IV) line in my arm or hand. Unfortunately, every time I got IV therapy it caused the left side of my body, from my shoulder to my toes, to go numb. For about an hour, I would get that tingly feeling you get when your foot falls asleep. No one could figure out why. The head of the oncology department had never experienced this with any other patient. Even with the tingling, the Broviac was worth it. But having the Broviac did mean I had tubes sticking out of my chest, and I had to have the dressing changed three times a week. It also meant I couldn't go swimming or do anything that would cause it to get wet.

Even though I had an IV line sticking out of my chest, I still had to get blood drawn the old-fashioned way each morning. Luckily, I had Larry as my phlebotomist. He didn't need to collect a lot of blood, so a finger prick was usually all that was needed. He learned very quickly I had poor circulation, partly due to genetics and partly due to the leukemia. Before he came into my room, he would wet a washcloth, stick it in the microwave to warm it up, and wrap my hand in the warm washcloth. This trick was a lifesaver as it got my blood circulating so he could easily get the amount of blood needed for the vial. I passed the trick on to every phlebotomist who came into my room. It's something I still do when I need blood work done.

While in the hospital, my Broviac was always attached to an IV. This made it difficult to wear regular shirts. I saw many younger children running around with no shirts or little tank tops, but I felt uncomfortable doing that as a thirteen-year-old girl. Luckily, my aunt found a pajama shirt with a wide neckline. It was perfect and allowed me to be covered while at the same time be comfortable having my Broviac accessed. Instead of the tubes being under my shirt and having to pull up my shirt every time a nurse needed to access my Broviac, the wide neckline allowed me to have the tubes come out the top and be on the outside of the shirt, making it easier for nurses to access it.

I stayed in the hospital for two weeks during my initial hospitalization. Due to the extreme pain the first week, my dad wanted me to have morphine, but he had to fight for it. The doctors were worried I would become addicted; Dad just wanted me to be comfortable. The protector side of my dad came out, and I remember him telling—not asking—the doctors to take me off over-the-counter pain medication and give me the strongest thing they could and to worry about addiction later.

It is amazing what two months of constant pain does to your psyche. I knew the leukemia caused my pain, and I knew I was being given morphine, but the nurses were unable to convince me the pain was already going away and would be gone forever in a couple of days when the chemotherapy started to work. They tried to get me to walk by forcing me to use the bathroom. I had been using a bedpan as it was more comfortable. (Seriously, who says a bedpan is more comfortable? You can imagine the severity of the pain I felt.) I pleaded with them to let me use the bedpan one last time and then I would walk. They made my mom leave the room as we argued this point because she would come to my defense. They finally agreed, and when I did get up to walk, I realized the pain was gone. I was able to move without pain, and I walked up and down the halls of the hospital as long as I could because it felt so good. I even discovered there was a beautiful fish tank down the hall near the elevators.

My first week in the hospital can only be described as a whirlwind experience. Everything happened so fast. Every day the nurses were coming in to tell us about a chemo I was taking or procedure I was going to have. To help with the chaos, my mom was given a binder and each medication or procedure had a corresponding sheet of paper, called Helping Hands. These papers described everything in terms anyone could understand. Each day my mom would get more and more Helping Hands and she would put them in the binder thinking she would read them later. I think my mom realized the seriousness of my diagnosis when the papers started piling up and she knew she hadn't read a single one. The binder was also a place to keep my test results, treatment plan, and all other important documentations related to my diagnosis. This was also a place my mom kept her own legal pad that she used to write down all her questions for the nurses and doctors, her to-do list, and her list of positive things that happened every day. Each night my mom and I would make a list of all the positive things that happened. Even on my worst days, we always found something good to be thankful for.

My mom spent many hours talking on the phone, answering the same questions over and over again with each call. The internet didn't exist back then, so there was no way of communicating with a large group of people at once. We didn't have too many visitors during this hospitalization. I was OK with that since I didn't have the energy for visits.

My best friend Sam threw me a surprise fourteenth birthday party that first week. My birthday was the first day Steven came to see me; it was awkward since neither of us knew what to say to each other. Theresa didn't come due to being away at college. Due to distance and weather (we were in the middle of a snowy Ohio winter), extended family didn't come to the hospital either.

Chemotherapy wreaks havoc on your body. It zaps

your energy and makes you nauseous. At home we had a puke bucket when we got sick. In the hospital, they give you these tiny kidney-shaped trays to puke in. All I could do was laugh; I didn't understand how they expected me to use something so small. Luckily, I got very good at knowing when I would get sick and found those little puke trays were quite handy.

My second week at the hospital, I got a roommate. Mary was younger than me and had a brain tumor. Her sister had already passed away from the same kind of brain tumor. Mary and her parents were able to help Mom and me cope with what was happening by telling us what to expect and where things were in the hospital. They also gave me a chance to realize things could be worse. Mary was the first cancer survivor I had ever met. She and her family lived with hope that Mary would survive, even though her sister had not.

Mary reminded me of the importance of having hope and to appreciate the good in every day: the good nurses who took their time to explain things to me; Father Ralko who would stop by daily with Communion and to talk; God; my parents; my stuffed dog Katie; and that my back pain was now gone!

4

STAFF WHO JUST DON'T GET IT

*U*nfortunately, not everyone who works in a children's hospital should work there. Some just don't understand what good bedside manners are. It was early in the morning, and I was sleeping when a man in a white coat entered my room stating, "Roll over. I need to put this cream on your back. I'm late for rounds." Being new to the whole hospitalization thing, I did what he told me. I rolled over and he quickly put cream on my back and left. He didn't tell me why he was putting cream on my back; he didn't explain what the cream was for; he didn't explain anything. I was extremely upset. I was terrified and had no idea what was about to happen to me.

We called Maria, my nurse practitioner, and asked her why some guy—we didn't know his name at the time—just came in, put cream on my back, and left. She explained the man was Frank, a resident, and I was going to have a spinal tap, and the cream was Emla cream. Emla cream numbs the area so I wouldn't feel the needle stick during the procedure. Until now I had been given local anesthesia to have a spinal tap or bone marrow biopsy done, so I hadn't

21

needed numbing cream. We explained to Maria that I wasn't comfortable with Frank doing my spinal tap. The way he had approached me made me nervous. First, it was a new procedure for me, and second, he had been rude. She told us she would do the procedure and not to worry, she would take care of him. Frank later came back telling me "it was time" (still not telling me what he was planning to do). Mom explained that Maria had already done the procedure. I could tell Frank was upset, but I didn't care.

My encounters with Frank were not over. He came to my room the next day to draw blood from my arm. I'm not sure why he and not a nurse or phlebotomist was taking my blood, but he did—or at least tried to. I explained he was to only take blood from my right arm, which was my preference. My bed was positioned against a wall on my right side. Instead of pulling the bed away from the wall, he told me to turn around in bed so my head was at the foot of the bed, giving him access to my right arm. I was still in severe pain at the time and turning in bed that way caused me a great deal of pain. I didn't question what he was doing because I was so new to this cancer world. I thought to myself, what an idiot, why would you have me turn around when you could just pull the bed from the wall? Then, he could not find a vein. I have small, rolling veins, and he kept poking and prodding to try to find one.

I was relieved when a nurse came in and told me I had to go for an echo and EKG. Frank told her I couldn't go because he had to get my blood. The nurse told him I *had* to go, and this wasn't an option. She said, he could get my blood when I got back to my room. I didn't know what an echo and EKG were, but I was happy to know I'd have a break from Frank hurting me.

When I got back from the procedures, Frank was

waiting for me, but so was my nurse. Apparently, Mom talked to my nurse while I was gone, and when I got back the nurse told Frank she would be drawing my blood, not him. The nurse pulled my bed from the wall and quickly found a vein. She didn't have enough vials, so she told Frank to get three 3cc vials. When he came back, he had the wrong size vial. The nurse turned to him and said in a very authoritative voice, "Go get them and don't come back until you find them." When he finally returned with the right size vial, he was in a terrible mood. Again, I thought to myself, you're an idiot. There was a four-inch-long black and blue mark on my arm from where he tried and failed to get my blood. That was the last time I saw Frank. To this day, I don't let residents touch me with a needle.

The echo and EKG I received that day taught me a valuable lesson. This was the first time getting these tests and I didn't know what to expect, but I was happy to get away from Frank, so I didn't care what they were. My nurse walked with Mom as she pushed my wheelchair to the cardiology department to have the procedures done. Everywhere I went my IV pole went with me, as I was always attached to it. When we got there, I was put in a dark room and told to lie on the table. There was a TV in the room, and the nurse put the movie *Free Willy* on for me to watch. I got the echo first. The nurse squeezed warm goo on my chest and used a wand to take an ultrasound of my heart. I didn't like the goo as it was messy and got all over my clothes and me. Next came the EKG. The nurse doing the procedure stuck what looked like heart stickers all over my chest and then attached cables to each sticker. She struggled to get a reading from the stickers. She disconnected the cables and reattached the heart stickers multiple times, but nothing worked. I didn't mind as I was enjoying watching the movie.

After a couple of attempts, she finally called in another nurse for assistance. The second nurse immediately realized that she had been using stickers meant for babies. Since baby skin is so sensitive, these stickers weren't as sticky and didn't have the connection needed for my skin. The second nurse got the appropriate stickers and she was able to complete the procedure. I learned three things that day: first, children's hospitals are great because you get to watch movies during procedures; second, there is a difference between baby and children stickies for EKGs; and third, an echo and EKG should not take an hour and a half to complete.

During my initial hospitalization, a psychologist came to talk to me about guided imagery and how I could use it to cope with procedures. My grandpa was sick at the time, and prior to my diagnosis, we thought he would die. So Heaven had been on my mind. When the psychologist asked me to think of a place I wanted to be, I quickly replied "Heaven." I'm sure this sent a red flag to her since I had only just been diagnosed, and now I was thinking of Heaven. She asked me to describe Heaven. I told her it was white. "What color white?" she wanted to know. I thought to myself, "What kind of question is that?" and replied, "white white." I then went on to tell her squirrels who get electrocuted while running across power lines were in Heaven too. Again, I was thinking of my grandpa. Behind their house were power lines that squirrels would run across, and I was always worried one would get electrocuted and die. I'm not sure what she thought, but we never talked about guided imagery again.

A few days later, my psychologist returned because she was worried I didn't know what time of day it was. I had been up until 2 a.m. the past couple of nights talking with nurses. My shades were drawn and there was no clock in my room. I simply answered with, "I know the *Price is Right* is on at 11:00 a.m., not 11:00 p.m., and my shades are drawn because my view is of a brick building." Before she left, she insisted on opening the window blinds. I thanked her for the amazing view of the brick building and all the dust landing on me from the blinds being opened. Apparently, no one had opened those blinds in a long time.

When she left, I closed the blinds and called a nurse to get new sheets since mine were now covered in dust. On a positive note, after that, housekeeping dusted the blinds every day.

While in the hospital, I became very close to Mom, and we continue to have a great relationship. She did almost everything for me. Doing things for me gave her something to do to pass the time. Mom always lived in a bubble, and this experience had burst her bubble. She was thrown into the world of the unknown with me. Mom was afraid to leave my room. It wasn't because she was worried about me; I think she was afraid she would get lost. She only ventured as far as the nurses' station and family lounge on the floor. This worried my social worker, my psychologist, and I think at times, my dad.

It wasn't until a neighbor came to have lunch that she learned where the cafeteria was. Up until this point she ate off my tray, finishing what I didn't eat. She reasoned that we paid for it and we weren't going to throw leftover food away.

My social worker and psychologist came up with a plan. It was a very stupid plan, and they would have realized it was stupid if they had taken the time to get to know us. They wanted Mom and me to sign an agreement stating we would spend thirty minutes of quality time together every day when we went home. They wanted us to play cards together or something else fun. They didn't want my mom doing things for me at home.

I understood they wanted me to do the things I could for myself once we got home, but they didn't realize that when we got home, my mom would have other things to do. They also suggested that if we didn't do our thirty minutes of quality time, my stuffed animals had to be removed from my bedroom. They knew I liked stuffed animals, but if they had taken the time to understand the depth of my obsession with stuffed animals, they would have realized it would have been easier to remove me from my room.

I had an *insane* number of stuffed animals. When we explained this to them, they suggested I have Katie, my stuffed dog, taken from me for a few hours, knowing she was important to me. I adamantly said no. I was not going to have them dictate when I could have her. Katie was my comfort; she was my sense of normalcy. I forget what punishment we finally agreed on. In the end, Mom and I signed the agreement to make them happy. Mom and I still laugh about our forced "quality time" agreement. When we got home, Mom continued to do things for me when I wasn't feeling well, but if I could, I would do things for myself. It was a way to feel normal again.

My most memorable and favorite social worker visit was when I was in the outpatient clinic. Brian joined my mom and me for this trip to the clinic. Brian was sitting in the waiting room, respecting my privacy while I had the chemo hooked up to my Broviac, and mom had run out to the car. I was in the treatment room alone when my social worker came to see me. I wasn't feeling well that day, and my social worker was the last person I wanted to see. I felt I was going to get sick, so I asked if she would get Brian and bring him back to the treatment room. Instead of doing what I asked, she proceeded to ask me how I knew Brian, who he was and other questions I was in no mood to answer. As my frustration grew, I finally yelled, "Go get Brian!" She quickly left and returned with him. I told Brian I was about to be sick as she just stood there continuing to ask me questions.

Then it happened. I got sick. I vomited all over the floor, taking aim at her shoes as she was standing directly in front of me. I was disappointed that I missed her shoes by a few inches. I didn't like my social worker when I was an inpatient, and I really didn't like her now. I had told her I wasn't feeling well, but she didn't care. She didn't need to know who Brian was, and if she had taken the time to get to know me during my initial hospitalization, she would have known. After that, I don't remember many more interactions with her.

Years later when I was in college, I took Social Work 101. On the first day, the teacher asked all of us why we were taking the course. The students around the room stated their reasons, most of which were to become a social worker. I simply replied that I wanted to know what social workers were supposed to do, since I didn't have a good one when I was in the hospital. I don't think the teacher liked my answer, but it was an honest one. I also took a course "How to Avoid Dying from Cancer." Yep, The Ohio State University *does* have a class on everything. I took it because it was a one-credit course and I thought it would be fun since I had already avoided dying from cancer.

I was completely surprised when I got my final grade: B. To this day, I laugh at getting a B when I should have received an A by default. I'm pretty sure I got the grade I did because many times during class I would raise my hand

and correct the teacher. The book we were using was out of date and I didn't want the other students to get the wrong information.

The bad staff I encountered taught me the importance of meeting a patient where they are. You can't go into a patient's room and expect them to know why you are putting cream on their back. You need to explain what the cream is and what it is used for. And if a patient has already accepted the fact they have cancer, why expect them to express grief and anger over it? Not everyone processes things the same way. Everyone's cancer journey is different. You need to figure out where the patient and families are in the process and use that as a starting point for helping them. Understanding this helped me become a better recreational therapist/child life specialist years later.

5

TREATMENT

$\mathcal{T}$he protocol they used to treat my cancer consisted of five phases, which lasted two and a half years. The first phase, induction, lasted five weeks and had the goal of getting me into remission. Then came consolidation, which lasted four to eight weeks, during which I received cranial radiation. This is when I lost my hair and felt the most nauseous. The next phase was interim maintenance, which lasted eight weeks, followed by another eight weeks of delayed intensification, and then maintenance, which lasted two years.

Even though everything was planned, treatments and/or phases were often delayed due to low blood counts or fevers. There were many times when my doctors had to lower the dosage of my chemotherapy because the full amount would drop my absolute neutrophil count (ANC) too low. ANC is a way to measure the status of a cancer patient's immune system and their risk of infection. The lower the ANC the higher the risk of infection. In order to receive chemotherapy, my ANC had to be 500 or higher. With my ANC frequently dropping below 500 and dosage of my chemotherapy being decreased, we asked the doctors if this would affect my chances of survival. They assured us everyone responds to chemotherapy differently and my body knows how much it needs and can take.

After my initial hospitalization, I went to the outpatient clinic to receive the majority of my treatment. On occasion, I would have to be hospitalized for a fever, low blood counts, or for a specific chemo drug. For the first six months, I returned to the outpatient clinic every Monday, Wednesday, and Friday. It became my home away from home for the next two and a half years. The outpatient clinic was located next to the inpatient unit on the fifth floor. I didn't mind going to clinic as I got to see all my nurses, who had become part of my family.

The waiting room was the biggest part of the clinic. It was a large, rectangular room with a TV in the corner and toys for children to play with. Mom and I would visit with other patients while we waited for my name to be called. Once they called me, I would go to a room that reminded me of a small closet without a door to have my vitals checked and blood drawn.

Afterwards, I would go to an exam room, where we would talk to the doctor, then to the treatment room. It was a big, square room, with five chairs, three on one side and two on the other, each separated by a curtain. Each chair had a small TV attached to it. This was where I would spend my day when I received chemo or blood products. It was easy to visit with the other patients since the chairs were so close together.

Toward the end of my treatment, the clinic was moved to a newer section of the hospital. It was a much larger clinic with much nicer chairs, toys, and exam rooms, but I missed the old clinic and the intimacy it provided.

My first outpatient clinic was when it finally hit me

how sick I was and how serious having leukemia was. It was the first time I truly realized this was my new life. It was the first time I saw other children, most of them younger than me, dealing with cancer too. It was the first time I saw kids in all stages of their treatment. Some were just beginning like me, and some were only there for their one-month, six-month or yearly follow-up appointments. I finally realized that Children's Hospital was going to be my home away from home for the next two and a half years.

We were originally told by the doctors that my mom would be able to return to teaching as soon as I started outpatient chemotherapy. I would be able to stay at home by myself and my mom would only need to take off a few hours each week to drive me to my appointments. After the first few outpatient clinic visits, when we realized how long clinic appointments really lasted, it became clear she was going to stay a nurse for a few more months.

No one tells you how long clinic appointments are going to be, and they do vary for everyone, but for me they were long. I would show up at 9:00 a.m. and wait to be called to have my vitals taken and blood drawn, since the whole appointment hinged on my blood counts. After my blood was drawn, I would wait until the results came back. When they were back, usually an hour later, I would find out whether I could get my chemo or if I needed a blood transfusion. My blood counts had to be just right to get chemo. If they were too low, I would be sent home or admitted to the hospital. My blood counts also revealed if I needed red blood cells, platelets, or a plasma transfusion.

I would meet with the doctor after the results came back, and they would tell me the plan for the day, then they would order the chemotherapy and/or blood products. I would return to the waiting room until they arrived. Once they arrived, I was taken to the treatment room. After settling in the treatment room, I would be hooked up to an IV and given my chemotherapy. The wait time for the chemotherapy to be finished varied—sometimes it took fifteen minutes and sometimes it took two hours. Because of the initial numbness in my left side when I received IVs, they had to run the fluids at a slower rate, which delayed things. Once the chemo was done, I would have fluids run through my IV to help flush the chemotherapy through my system.

More often than not, I would need a blood transfusion, which took another hour. On days when I needed to have a spinal tap, bone marrow biopsy, or other procedure done, I would have to wait longer. Sometimes the procedure had to be done prior to the chemotherapy; other times I could have it done after. The "quick trip" to the clinic was often an all-day affair. We would arrive at nine in the morning and leave around 4:00 p.m., sometimes later and sometimes sooner, but we never knew. This uncertainty prevented my mom from returning to work, but luckily her principal was willing to work with her and promised her job would be waiting for her the next school year.

I quickly learned to read my body and could predict what my blood counts would be and if I needed a blood transfusion. Platelets help prevent bruising, so if I saw bruises all over my body, I knew I would be getting platelets. If I was freezing and no one else was, I knew I would need blood. Knowing these things helped me estimate how long we would be in the clinic.

Mom and I discovered my dad would never be able to tolerate going to clinic appointments with me. The amount of time spent just waiting would have driven him crazy. I had to find ways to occupy my time. This was before cell phones, laptops, and portable DVD players. We would bring things to keep us busy—a coloring book, word search, my brother's Game Boy—but often I was too distracted and preferred to just observe what was going on in the waiting room. The younger children playing with the clinic toys entertained me. People watching became my favorite pastime.

One of my favorite memories with my mom was when we were sitting in the treatment room, I was hooked up to an IV, and we heard a mother a few chairs down from us tell her child she would gladly trade places with her. Mom turned to me and said, "There is no way I could ever trade places with you." I have laughed for years about this because who says that? What parent sees their child in pain and wouldn't trade places with them? My mom, that's who. I have only met one other person whose parent said the same thing. My mom went on to explain I was stronger than she was and that's why she wouldn't trade places with me. I sadly agreed with her and thanked her for her honesty.

Years later I found out she felt guilty about not wanting to trade places. I told her not to feel guilty; that day is one of my greatest memories and I love her more for saying what she did and the honesty behind it.

I had countless bone marrow biopsies and spinal taps during the first six months of treatment. These tests were to confirm the chemo was working and that my bone marrow and spinal fluid were clear of leukemia cells. During one phase I had weekly spinal taps, with the occasional intrathecal chemotherapy. On these days I would have IT methotrexate administered directly into the spinal fluid during a spinal tap. Spinal taps were hard enough, but having chemo injected into your spinal fluid was not a fun experience; thankfully, the odd stinging feeling it caused didn't last long.

The hardest clinic days and the ones I dreaded the

most were the days I had to have a spinal tap and bone marrow biopsy on the same day. Neither procedure was enjoyable to begin with, and to have them on the same day made it worse. I would always have the spinal tap first. I would sit up and hunch over a pillow for that one. Immediately after, I would lay on my stomach to have the bone marrow biopsy. I would go home with my back and hip hurting. Thankfully, there were only a handful of days in which these procedures occurred on the same day as part of my treatment. I learned to love EMLA cream, as it made these procedures much more tolerable.

Cytoxan was one chemotherapy medication I had to receive as an inpatient. The drug was one of the more toxic medications and I would have to receive Lasix to clear my kidneys immediately after to prevent kidney damage. Taking medications like Cytoxan made me wonder what I really was doing to my body. My nurses came into my room in special chemotherapy gowns and gloves (think hazmat suit) to administer Cytoxan. Once my medication was hooked up to my IV, I was free to do what I wanted until the Cytoxan bag was empty. My mother and I decided to go sit by the fish tank we had found previously in the lobby.

My first experience with Lasix was a memorable one. My nurse found us at the fish tank and let me know she was going to hook up the Lasix and that it would make me have to go to the bathroom. I asked if I would have enough time to get back to my room. I had to use the toilet in my room, as they had a special bowl, called a "hat," placed in the toilet to catch and measure my urine output. She assured me I would have enough time because Lasix takes a bit of time to take effect.

Boy, was she wrong! It took effect immediately. I was running back to my room with my IV pole in tow barely making it to the bathroom in time. When they say Lasix makes you pee, they aren't kidding. I sat on the toilet for an hour, only getting up when the hat was full. I was amazed there was that much fluid inside me. As I sat on the toilet, I was jealous of boys who could remain in bed and use a urinal. Being a girl and having Lasix was not fun.

Another obstacle preventing my mom from returning to work was my insatiable appetite. I was on a high dose of prednisone, which caused me to eat and eat and eat. When I say eat, I mean it. One day my mom and I wrote down everything I ate in a day: a box of Noodle Roni, a bag of popcorn, a turkey sandwich, a bowl of pretzels, three bowls of puffed rice, two English muffins, a container of cherry tomatoes, carrots and dip, a whole pizza, a box of macaroni and cheese and a can of chicken noodle soup!

There were times when someone brought over dinner for my whole family, but I would eat the entire meal, so Mom had to cook for herself, my dad, and my brother. By the time she was done making them dinner, I would be hungry again. One night a friend ordered a large pizza for the family, and I ended up eating the whole thing by myself. I was amazed because before it would have taken me an entire week to eat that much food. It was good that I was eating so much as I had lost twenty pounds since being diagnosed and only weighed eighty pounds.

I loved this part of my treatment: I could eat anything I wanted, and I didn't gain too much weight. I went through a stage where each night at around 11:00 p.m., while watching *Rescue 911* on TV, I would eat a block (half to three-quarters of a pound) of Muenster cheese. Yep, *half a pound* of cheese! After I finished the cheese I would go to bed. This lasted for a month or two. Since I felt I was eating like a pig, my grandma gave me a stuffed pig. I named it Prednisone Pig, after the steroid that caused me to eat so much.

I eventually became addicted to the prednisone. This was the only medication I enjoyed taking and craved. Instead of my mom telling me it was time to take it, I was telling her. My body needed it. When it came time to taper me off the steroid, I went through withdrawal. Instead of wanting to eat everything, I had no desire to eat anything. I had lost my insatiable appetite. When this happened, I was in the hospital and they wouldn't discharge me home until I ate. My mom encouraged me to start eating again one grape at the time. We had to record what I was eating to show the doctors I was eating enough.

Even though I had started eating, I wasn't eating enough in the doctor's eyes, so my mom fudged the list of what I ate so I could go home, knowing I would probably eat better at home. Once home, I slowly regained my appetite.

Thankfully, only some of the chemotherapy made me nauseous. My glucose went up for a short period of time, forcing me to eliminate sugar from my diet, but that didn't affect me too much since I didn't eat a lot of sugar anyway. Although, would you believe, I craved apple pie more than anything at that time. A friend of the family was nice enough to find a sugar-free apple pie for me.

One chemotherapy drug caused my urine to be red. The funny part is my nurse forgot to tell me this, and when I went to the bathroom, I thought I was bleeding and yelled for her. She quickly explained it was a common side effect and I shouldn't worry. I told her that would have been nice to know *before* I went to the bathroom.

On my first visit to radiology, I had my mask made. The technician took a mold of my head and used it to make the mask. The mask was used to protect parts of my brain. They marked the exact spot for the radiation on the mask instead of my skin. Then the mask attached to the table, preventing me from moving my head during radiation therapy.

The technician making the mask explained that they make the masks less scary for kids by decorating them to look like animals. They asked if I wanted my mask decorated. I said sure and asked for it to look like a German Shepherd. I think they were expecting something easier, but they were up to the challenge. The next day I had a German Shepherd mask. I never told the technicians I thought it looked like a kangaroo. I appreciated their efforts in making me more comfortable with radiation by doing fun, silly things like decorating a mask.

The hardest time for me was having chemotherapy and radiation at the same time. I got extremely nauseous. We would keep a puke bucket in the car in case I felt sick after clinic appointments. Luckily for me, there was an anti-nausea drug called Zofran. I called Zofran a miracle pill because it worked so well at preventing me from getting nauseous.

The worst side effect I experienced was from the chemotherapy vincristine. I developed the "vincristine walk," which causes you to walk toe-heel, as if you were prancing, instead of the usual heel-toe. It also hurt to walk, so I walked very slowly. When I first started walking like this, my parents were worried I would need physical therapy to learn how to walk properly again. When I went to see my doctor, before I could even show him the funny way I was walking, he was demonstrating it. He explained it was a common side effect and in time I should start walking normally again. He also advised that I become a couch potato while on vincristine, because it could cause long-term damage to my joints. I took advantage of the fact my doctor told me to be a couch potato. I did as little physical activity as I could. For months I had the "vincristine walk." I had to concentrate if I wanted to walk normally. I could only walk upstairs one step at a time.

Then one night around midnight, on my way to bed, I suddenly realized I could walk normally again. The "vincristine walk" disappeared as quickly as it had come. Since I had not been able to walk normally for months, I walked around the house for an hour. I woke up my dad to show him I could walk. I had never been so grateful. It is so easy to take something as simple as walking for granted. It is so easy to take *life* for granted. This was another experience reminding me to not take anything for granted, to cherish the gifts God has given us, and to remain hopeful.

Mouth sores are a common side effect for anyone taking chemotherapy. To prevent this, I was given two kinds of mouthwash to take multiple times a day. Both mouthwashes were disgusting. I used the mouthwash during my first hospitalization, but after that I stopped taking it as did many other teenagers. I knew my risk of developing mouth sores increased, but I didn't care. Not having to taste the mouthwash was worth the risk. Thankfully, I never developed the mouth sores my doctors warned me about.

The medicine I hated the most and dreaded taking was Bactrim. I called it a horse pill because the pill was gigantic compared to all the others. I couldn't swallow pills that were much smaller than this one, so I didn't even try swallowing Bactrim. Mom tried mixing it in Kool-Aid, but it tasted disgusting. I could tolerate all my other medications, but not this one. Eventually, the anxiety of taking Bactrim got the best of me and I would get sick just thinking about taking it. Mom decided to ignore the doctor's directives; it wasn't a chemo drug, just a preventative medication, so she saw no harm in not taking it. The benefits of taking it did not outweigh the costs. I was relieved, and we didn't tell anyone.

About a month later I ended up in the hospital with pneumonia. I was hospitalized for three weeks; the x-rays of my lungs looked like clouds. The odd thing is I felt fine. Other than a cough, I didn't feel any chest pain. My doctors were shocked, and they kept asking me if it felt like I had an elephant sitting on my chest while I breathed. After a week, I was transferred to the Pediatric Intensive Care Unit (PICU). My x-rays looked so bad they were worried they were going to have to intubate me to help me breathe. They wanted to be ready if and when it did happen.

What amazes me the most is that I remember going to the PICU, and I remember waking up a week later in an isolation room on the fifth floor (the hematology/oncology floor). I never had to be intubated, yet I have no memories of that week at all. When I woke up, I asked my mom what happened in the PICU. She was confused by the question because she told me nothing happened. I asked her if I was asleep the whole time. Again, she was confused because she told me that I ate, got out of bed, visited with people, and received Communion from Father Ralko every day. I was in disbelief when she told me I did all those things. I had no memory of doing anything. I somehow missed a whole week of my life!

When my doctors found out we had stopped taking Bactrim, they were upset at my mom because Bactrim helps prevent infections, including pneumonia. They made my mom feel guilty until a nurse told her the type of pneumonia I had would not have been prevented by Bactrim. As a result, my doctors prescribed the liquid form of Bactrim for me.

Later that day, my nurse walked into my room with the liquid Bactrim in a syringe. I asked her what it tasted like, something I always asked, especially on medications that were preventative. She laughed, and my mom offered to try a pencil eraser–size drop of it. She immediately gagged and spit it out in a tissue. Mom described liquid Bactrim as a thick, white substance that was bitter and chalky. Even after eating a bowl of Lucky Charms, she could still taste the chalkiness. My mom told the nurse she should try it because no child should ever take this. My nurse did and had the same reaction as my mom. She then turned to me and said, "Carolyn, you're not taking this. It is the most disgusting thing I ever tasted. There is no way you could take three cc's of this when I couldn't tolerate a drop. Your mom is right. No one should take this." Mom suggested she call the pharmacist and have him taste it. He did, agreed with the nurse, and pulled it from the shelf.

Since neither the pill nor liquid form of Bactrim was an option for me, I was prescribed pentamidine, which is an inhaled medication using a nebulizer. Once a month, I would go to the respiratory clinic for my treatment. This was a much better option, one that in my opinion they should offer all children, inhaling pentamidine once a month was worlds better than swallowing a horse pill daily.

As I progressed through my protocol, I went to clinic less and less until I was only going once a year. I learned a lot during my hospitalizations, clinic trips, and talking with other cancer patients.

My experience taught me it's OK to play the cancer card, not all chemo makes you sick, and Zofran is an amazing drug. Radiation and chemo are a bad combination. Losing your hair is fun and it doesn't hurt when it falls out. If a nurse gives you Lasix, make sure you're close to the bathroom and plan to spend an hour there. If you have poor circulation, warm your hand under hot water or wrap it in a warm washcloth before a finger stick. Patients have rights too. If you ask a doctor if it will hurt, the typical response is, "You may feel pressure" or "It might sting." Some chemo makes your taste buds change, causing everything to taste metallic. Your sense of smell might become that of a bloodhound. Not everyone survives, you will make friends and a couple of months later you may be attending their funeral. It's OK to hate cancer one minute and feel it was a blessing the next.

Many people would think having leukemia would be a terrible thing, but I saw it as a blessing. Even with the medical mistake, the horrible-tasting chemotherapy, the resident with no bedside manners, and a social worker and psychologist who didn't take the time to get to know me, I would do it all over again because I am thankful for what cancer has taught me.

Six years later, I wrote "My Days" as a remembrance of how I spent 1994. It was a time in my life when I was so weak and vulnerable but felt safe and strong at the same time.

My Days

Hospital visits Monday, Wednesday, Friday.
Blood transfusions, Spinal Taps, Chemo,
Needles, Pills, Procedures,
Doctors, Nurses, Patients, Parents.
Nowhere to run, nowhere to hide.
I had to keep fighting so I would survive.
So many new concepts, so many new things
A new way of life, a new way to live.
No more going out, only staying in,

41

No more school only trips to Children's.
I found a new family of friends,
I soon longed for the days I spent with them.
I miss the long days I sat all day
On those Mondays, Wednesdays, Fridays.

6

GOD WORKS IN MYSTERIOUS WAYS

*F*our months after my diagnosis, I had a Friday off. I was excited to have the day off where I didn't have a clinic appointment and I could stay home. Then I developed a fever of 101 degrees. It wasn't my first fever, but it would turn out to significantly impact my life. Mom and I held off as long as we could before going the hospital. When you have cancer, you follow the "Fever Rule." Any fever over 100 degrees is a serious fever and you must be admitted for observation. My day off was cancelled. There we were, once again being admitted to the hospital. Once I was admitted, blood cultures were taken to try to determine the cause of my fever and my nurse started administering broad-spectrum antibiotics through my Broviac catheter.

Throughout my cancer treatment I watched everything that was happening to me. That day and throughout the weekend I noticed a pulsing in the IV line, something I had never seen before. I asked each nurse on every shift why it was pulsing, and each nurse thought nothing of it. I wanted an answer because in the past four months, I had never seen my IV line pulsing. I was very aware this was something different and I wanted to know why.

What happened next I can only attribute to another miracle. Monday morning, Linda was supposed to be in a meeting, but it was cancelled, allowing her to come to work. She was one of the nurses who genuinely enjoyed having me as a patient, and when she saw I was in the hospital, she wanted to be the one taking care of me. When she came to check on me, I asked her about the pulsing in the line. Linda was there when I was diagnosed and remembered three seemingly disconnected facts: one, that my blood would not clot when the Broviac was originally placed; two, that my body went numb with every IV; and three, the tests that had been done never revealed why I had a fever and why my fever would not go away, even though I was given a battery of antibiotics to kill everything. She was able to connect the dots.

She explained the pulsing was most likely caused by my heartbeat, but that it should not be doing that. She suspected my Broviac wasn't in the right place, but the doctors disagreed. She really stood up for me and argued with them to get an x-ray taken. When the results of the x-ray came back, it showed nothing wrong with the placement of the Broviac. My doctors wanted to send me home on antibiotics, but Linda was still not convinced, especially since there was still no cause for my high fever or pulsing IV line. She would not sign my release papers until the doctors ordered one more test and proved to her that everything was safe. My doctors were not happy, but they ordered a blood gas test anyway.

Linda was right: The blood gases were from arterial blood, not venous. My Broviac had been placed in an artery, instead of a vein where it should have been. Once the mistake was discovered, my fever broke and never returned.

The Broviac being in an artery explained the excessive bleeding the day the Broviac was placed, the left-sided numbness (the doctors now believed the fluid going through the IV was hitting a nerve and causing the tingling sensation), and the pulsing in the line. My doctors and nurses were surprised I hadn't experienced any complications such as a blood clot or stroke due to the misplaced Broviac.

I'm a firm believer the excessive bleeding, tingling, and pulsating IV line were signs from God. He was trying to show us my central line was in the wrong spot, but God doesn't fix man-made problems. God only guides man to find the problems and fix them. He sends us living angels to do the work for Him. My fever put me in the hospital and Linda's meeting being cancelled allowed her to be my nurse. These two events allowed Linda to put all the pieces together and discover my medical mistake. May 9th, God sent me Linda, she's my living angel.

Surgery was scheduled for the next day to replace my Broviac. I wasn't happy with the news. I didn't want to spend one more day in the hospital, especially since I was feeling fine now that my fever had disappeared. I begged my doctors to allow me to go home—all I wanted to do was to see Misty. My doctor finally agreed to a couple of hours' leave of absence. They knew it would do me good to go home to see my dog.

The scariest part of the discovery was knowing all the chemotherapy I had been given intravenously had gone straight to my heart before being circulated through my veins, instead of the other way around like it was supposed to. We asked if this would cause damage to my heart. My doctors assured me my heart was fine.

People often asked if we sued the hospital, but my family and I chose not to. Why? Because everyone makes mistakes. Luckily, I didn't have any complications or long-term effects, and the second Broviac worked perfectly.

I believe my medical mistake is an example of God working in mysterious ways. Some might say it was a coincidence, but I think otherwise. Why? Because everything had a purpose and reason for happening. God knew my Broviac was placed in an artery, God knew He needed to create signs for it to be discovered, and God sent me Linda. He had a plan the minute there was a problem. As much faith as we have in God, He has the same faith in us.

7

CONTROL

When I was diagnosed with cancer, I felt I had lost all control over my life. For months I had been controlled by pain, and now pills and protocols controlled me. I didn't have a choice. At fourteen years old you are looking for autonomy, you are looking to break away from your parents, and you start figuring out who you are. I skipped this developmental stage or at least feel it was delayed.

Cancer took away my freedom to make choices. I had to take the chemotherapy or I would die. I had to go to the outpatient clinic three days a week for the chemotherapy or I wouldn't get better. I had to stop going to school and being around my classmates or I would get sick. I had to rely on people to help me because I was too weak or sick. I should have been figuring out who I was and becoming more independent. Instead, I was becoming a teenage cancer survivor.

When you don't have control over your life, you try to find every little way to take some control back. Being fourteen in a children's hospital has its challenges. There are very few patients your age, so almost everything is geared toward a child. I figured I might as well befriend the nurses and embrace the childlike atmosphere I was in.

I have always been a child at heart, as evidenced by my love of stuffed animals. I also embrace a playfulness with those I am closest to. This personality trait carried over to how I coped with being sick. Some might say I acted like a baby, but I would disagree; I was just finding a way to cope with what was happening and the environment I was in. I was a fourteen-year-old girl who loved stuffed animals, who was away from home, who had just been told she had leukemia, and who had entered a world full of unknowns. Could I have dealt with it better? Of course, but I dealt with it the best way I knew how.

As I have already said, I didn't know how to swallow pills. I didn't take the liquid form of my medication for two reasons. First, many of my chemotherapy drugs did not come in liquid form. Second, those that did tasted worse than a crushed pill in Kool-Aid. I couldn't swallow a pill no matter how hard I tried, and going from never having to take medicine to taking multiple pills per day is a major challenge for anyone.

For those reading who cannot swallow a pill, I discovered it's a mental thing. No matter how hard you try, you may never be able to swallow pills. My nurses tried to teach me to put the pill in the back of my mouth and quickly swallow a large gulp of water by tilting my head back. That didn't work for me. I practiced with mini M&Ms and could easily swallow those but couldn't swallow the pill.

It is often suggested to mix pills in with your child's favorite food. Bad idea—your child's favorite food will quickly become a food they hate, and why take something they love away?

Since I couldn't swallow pills, my mom crushed them and mixed them with Kool-Aid, and after thirty minutes of stirring (I had the best mom ever for doing that), I would take the shot of Kool-Aid. (By the way, I won't drink Kool-Aid anymore.) I took the control I needed by mentally preparing myself to take the pill. I knew the crushed medicine was sufficiently stirred after a few minutes, but I needed thirty to prepare myself. My mom got a lot of flak for this, but she did it because she knew I needed it and it gave her an excuse to sit down and relax for thirty minutes. I'm willing to do anything, but I must mentally prepare myself first.

Another way I took control was by having fun with my nurses, although I'm pretty sure they didn't always enjoy it. Whenever a nurse came in and told me she had pills I needed to take, I would do one of two things. I would hide them somewhere in my room when she turned her back. I had been given a stuffed Kanga from Winnie the Pooh whose pouch was a perfect hiding spot, and I would make the nurses play the Hot and Cold game; once they found where I hid the medicine, I would take it. Or I would tell the nurse she had to come back in half an hour.

This often annoyed the student nurses because they had to watch me take my medicine. I would tell them they could watch me take it when they came back in thirty minutes. They eventually figured out they needed to come to my room thirty minutes *before* they wanted me to take the meds knowing I would stall, but I always took my medication when I said I would.

Both "games" I played were my way of taking control and giving myself time to get ready to take the medicine. I had great nurses and amazing doctors who were compassionate and grew to understand my need for control.

I eventually learned to hide the pill in a piece of

banana. Surprisingly, the large piece of banana was easier to swallow even though it was bigger than the pill. Years later, I discovered the banana thing was a bad idea because when I took a bite, I would automatically swallow it. I had to retrain my body to chew the piece of banana.

Another way I took control was with my stuffed dog Katie. I have no idea when or where I got Katie, but I had her for years. I'm guessing I got her in the first grade shortly after we had to euthanize our German Shepherd named Katie. Even though I was fourteen years old, Katie came with me to every procedure, every surgery (at a children's hospital they let you bring your stuffed animals into the surgery room), every trip to the hospital, and every outpatient clinic visit. Again, some might say this was childish, but I still slept with stuffed animals, so why would my love of stuffed animals change just because I had cancer?

During each procedure, no matter if it was a simple finger prick or something more complicated like a bone marrow biopsy, I clutched Katie. She helped me control my emotions. If I was scared, I would hug her. If I needed to cry, I would use her fur to wipe my tears away. Two and a half years later, when I was at the tail end of my treatment and I was sixteen years old, Katie still came with me to the hospital. She was my comfort, she was my support, and she made everything all right.

When I had to have emergency surgery to replace the Broviac, I planned to take Katie to surgery with me. To ensure the right stuffed animal gets back to the right child (since they remove the animal as soon as the child is asleep), they put an identification band with the child's name on the stuffed animal's paw. When it came time to give Katie an identification band, I insisted she have one with "Katie Koncal" on it. To me, Katie was a real animal, just like in *The Velveteen Rabbit*, when the rabbit becomes a real rabbit because he is loved so much. That is what Katie was to me, my Velveteen Dog.

As I was heading into surgery, one of the nurses asked me what my stuffed cat's name was. I was upset and offended he called Katie a cat. She looked like a dog; she had a long nose and long floppy ears and, in my mind, didn't resemble a cat at all. I asked the nurse to apologize to Katie for calling her a cat. He looked at me and at another nurse and stated, "I'm not apologizing to a stuffed animal." I quickly replied, "I'm not going into surgery until you do." The second nurse, recognizing the seriousness in my voice and knowing the importance of me getting into surgery on time, said, "Just apologize," and so he did.

Looking back on that moment, I was taking control. I do feel bad about taking some of that nurse's dignity away, but hopefully, he learned a lesson—stuffed animals are very important to those who have them.

Using my voice was also a way I took control. I voiced my concern about my hesitation to take pills. Although some nurses didn't like the way I did this, eventually they gave me the control I needed. I asked questions about what was going on around me and to me. I talked to my doctors during procedures. During spinal taps, since I couldn't see behind me, I always asked, "Am I dripping yet?" meaning was the spinal fluid flowing. This gave me reassurance and a time frame of how much longer the procedure would last. They would tell me when each vial was filled, providing me with a little more control during the procedure.

I used my voice to control conversations. By sharing my experience with others, I realized people were genuinely interested in learning about my leukemia but didn't know what to ask. I took the first step and mentioned cancer; I said the dreaded word first. As soon as the "elephant in the room" was acknowledged, people became more comfortable around me. People make many assumptions when you have cancer. My favorites were "Shouldn't you be dead?" or "Are you going to die?" I always laughed when people asked me those questions because I loved the honesty. By laughing about it and explaining that not all cancers are death sentences, I was able to educate people as well.

In high school I discovered why so many people asked me if I was going to die. When I had to write a paper on leukemia for health class, I realized every book in the school library was out of date. Not a single book stated leukemia was a survivable cancer. I notified the school librarian and she discarded all those books. I didn't realize it then, but I was part of the earliest generation where surviving cancer was more common than dying from it.

I could not control what others thought of me, but I could control how I responded. A few kids voiced their opinions. One girl, whom I had been classmates with since the first grade, called me "leukemia girl." When I heard what she had called me, I went up to her at a football game and asked if it was true. I told her it was OK to call me leukemia girl because I was a girl and I had leukemia. I just asked that if she was going to call me that, she do it to my face instead of behind my back. She quickly turned and walked away. I know people joked and laughed at me, and it hurt, but in the end, if someone was going to make fun of me, I didn't want or need that person as a friend.

One nurse learned how to use my sense of control against me. Every week there was an inpatient support group, and when I was hospitalized, I was encouraged to go. I hated going because I was the oldest one in the group and couldn't relate to the other kids. The nurse who ran the group soon realized that if she could convince another patient, who was a cute teenage boy, to go to the support group, I would also go. The support group always ended with a group hug, so sitting next to Josh meant I got a hug from him. She knew it was my choice to attend the support group, but she used the fact I thought he was cute to sway my choice.

Control allowed me to understand and become comfortable with what was happening to me. I knew my nurses, my medications, the various procedures—nothing was new anymore. Then halfway through my treatment, my dad lost his job and I got angry. How was he supposed to afford college for my sister and brother and treatment for me? Did they terminate him because my medical bills were so high? Being the financial guy he was, Dad made it work and we all survived, but I was still angry. I knew things were going to change and I knew the comfort zone I was in would soon disappear; unfortunately, I had no control over it.

My dad losing his job had a huge impact on my treatment because our health insurance changed. I now had to go to a health maintenance organization (HMO) to get my weekly blood work instead of having it done at Children's Hospital. I hated this. I had grown comfortable with the nurses at Children's and I knew how they did things, how they drew blood or inserted an IV without it hurting. I didn't like the nurses at the HMO, and I didn't like the lack of control. I didn't like being forced to go there by some insurance company, and I especially didn't like the way they drew my blood and never could get my results to Children's in a timely manner.

Per my protocol, I had been going to the Children's Hospital outpatient clinic every Friday for chemotherapy and would have my blood taken and tested prior to the chemotherapy to ensure my blood counts were high enough to receive it. During this time, most of my blood draws at Children's Hospital were done through finger pricks; they didn't need a lot of blood, so they saw no reason to draw from a vein. They knew the warm-the-hand trick Larry had taught me and had no problem waiting an extra three to five minutes while I warmed up my hand, since they knew they would get a better blood flow. Once they pricked my finger and saw I was bleeding, they would tap the vial against the drop of blood, never touching my finger with the vial. This was a pain-free way of doing finger pricks. On occasion, depending on the tests ordered, they would draw my blood from a vein, and I knew which tests required a larger amount of blood to be drawn.

When I went to the HMO, I went early in the week, on a Monday or Tuesday, knowing they would have plenty of time to fax the results to Children's Hospital for my Friday appointment. When I walked into the lab for the first time, they immediately asked to see my arms. I asked why, and they said that's how they take blood from someone my age. I quickly responded, "No you're not, you're taking it from my finger!" I knew they only needed a small amount of blood and didn't need a vein in my arm. They said they didn't do finger pricks for teenagers and I adamantly stated, "I don't care what you do for other teenagers, you are only pricking my finger!" I told them they could look at the veins in my arms, but they couldn't touch them. I then told them it wasn't my choice to go there, and if they were going to take my blood, they were going to do it the way Children's Hospital did it and that was through a finger prick.

They finally relented. I informed them I needed to warm my hand and explained why. The look I got from the phlebotomist was horrific. You would have thought I had asked her to commit murder when all I was asking for was three to five minutes to warm up my hand under hot water. When it came time to draw my blood, she pricked my finger, waited for me to bleed, then took the vial and with each drop scraped the vial against my finger, causing me pain.

I was already mad I was there and now they were causing me unnecessary pain. So I did what I needed to do. I spoke up, explaining how Children's Hospital pricked my finger and the painless way of tapping the vial against the drop of blood. I asked if she would stop scraping the tip of my finger across the vial, but the phlebotomist just looked at me.

Arguing about finger pricks vs. needle sticks went on for weeks, until finally, they put a standing order in my chart for finger pricks, although they hated waiting for me to warm up my hand. One day when I was in the waiting room at the HMO, I noticed all children and teenagers were offered a sucker or sticker after their labs were drawn, something I had never been offered. I then heard a nurse around the corner say, "You can have her." Next thing I knew, my name was called, and I realized they had been talking about me. I became incredibly angry. I knew the nurses in the lab didn't like me and I was OK with that because I didn't like them either, but this showed *how* much they didn't like me. So, I did the only thing I could think of that made me happy. I entered the lab room with the mentality that the more I aggravated the phlebotomist, the happier I was when I left. Each visit I took a little extra time warming up my hand, and I always reminded them that Children's Hospital did it better.

Another thing I had no control over was that the HMO would never fax my lab results to Children's Hospital on time. Each Friday, I would show up for my appointment at the Children's outpatient clinic only to be told I had to wait because my doctors had to call the HMO and get my results before I could get the chemo. When I questioned the HMO about the delay, their response was "sometimes it takes longer to get your results back." I didn't accept the excuse because I knew for a fact they could get my results in an hour if they wanted to, and four days was plenty of time. Eventually, with enough complaining from my family and me, and pushing from my doctors at Children's, my insurance company agreed I could go back to getting my blood drawn at Children's Hospital. I regained control of my treatment and was happy to say goodbye to the HMO.

During my entire treatment and into adulthood, another form of control was not allowing nurses to draw blood from or to insert an IV into my left arm. Everything had to be done in my right arm. This was a mental thing for me. I didn't want to jerk away, and I felt that I could control my right arm better than my left. I always allowed the nurses to look at my left arm, I do have a good vein there, but I never let them use it.

In 2007, I decided to conquer the fear of no needles on the left side of my body by getting a tattoo on my left ankle. It reads January 24–25, 1994, with a cross and wraps around my ankle. It symbolizes the day I went into the hospital, the day I was diagnosed, and that God was with me. I'm glad I did it, but I discovered getting a tattoo over your ankle bone and Achilles tendon is very painful, so if you don't like pain, I don't recommend those areas.

Since then, I have gotten more tattoos, each one reminding me of what I have been through. A dove on my right scapula symbolizes the peace I found after dealing with depression, and a turtle on my left scapula symbolizes strength. If you are considering getting a tattoo, there are two things you should know. First, it's permanent, so get something you will want on your body fifty or sixty years from now. Second, they are addicting, so be prepared to feel the need to get more.

Knowing that control is important to children helped me when I worked as a recreational therapist/child life specialist at a children's hospital many years later. Many times I had to let the child feel as if they were in control before they would trust me.

With one three-year-old, I would go in to play with her every day, and every day she would hide under her sheets. After a few times of visiting her and talking to her while she was hiding, she peeked out from under the sheets. I saw she had stuffed animals—a dog and a cat. I picked them up and had them chase each other. I barked and meowed the entire time. Before I knew it, she reached out and grabbed the cat and meowed while she chased the dog I had. This continued for a while and was the first time she showed she trusted me, and it was because I had the patience to wait and let her feel in control of the play session. The next day she was out in the common area playing on a computer. I had just sat down next to her when her nurse stopped by to give her a mouse sticker for being so good when she got her blood drawn earlier. She took the sticker and gave it to me. The mouse sticker she gave me meant the world to me. I knew my patience truly had paid off.

Another time, I had two patients who both carried stuffed animals around with them, Sage, a dog and Gunther, a hippo. Neither child would express how they felt when asked. One day I decided to ask the stuffed animals how they felt and, believe it or not, they responded. For the entire therapy session that day, I didn't once speak to the child, only to the stuffed animal.

Later, in an interdisciplinary meeting, I told the team how the children felt, and everyone was surprised the children had opened up to me. I told them they hadn't, but their stuffed animals had. I was able to get the information I needed by allowing the children to be in control.

Having control when you're going through cancer treatment or any other life-changing event is crucial. I'm sure my nurses didn't appreciate the inconvenience of having to play the Hot or Cold game or having to come back in thirty minutes to watch me take my pills. But the good nurses understood. The good nurses knew giving me the perception of control made me an easier patient.

8

FAMILY

*N*ot only did my life change when I was diagnosed with cancer, but my family's lives did too, especially my mom's. She became more than just a mother to me. She took a leave of absence from being a music teacher to become my personal nurse. She ensured I got my medication and learned how to change my dressings, although she wasn't very good at it. She would answer the phone in the middle of changing my dressing. I would yell at her, telling her my dressing change was more important than a phone call. She stayed with me at the hospital during inpatient treatment, drove me to the clinic three times a week for outpatient chemotherapy, comforted me when I was sick, helped me fall asleep by saying the rosary, and slept on the floor in my bedroom when I needed her to. She tolerated my mood swings and understood they were caused by the medication. She entertained me when I was bored and cooked for me when I had an insatiable appetite due to steroids. She wiped my tears away when I cried and celebrated each day with me.

Soon after my diagnosis, my friends went on with their

lives, leaving me feeling alone and isolated. Mom stepped in and took their place and became my best friend. She was there for me when others left. The journey we took together that year brought us closer and allowed us to see a side of each other we would never have seen if not for my cancer. Later, we realized we had placed ourselves in our own box to shield us from anything or anyone else.

My dad played a big part in my care as well. I think my diagnosis shocked him. I mean, nobody ever wants to hear your child has cancer. He realized there was nothing he could do but "go with the flow," hoping and praying the doctors could make his daughter healthy again. He was very interested in which procedures I was having and what kind of medications I was on. When I was first hospitalized and during every hospitalization after, he would come to my hospital room after work and read the newspaper. We didn't talk much, but his presence was enough. I didn't realize it then, but that was his way of caring, his way of showing me support.

When I got home, he also relinquished the family room and his favorite chair to me, so I would be more comfortable. I may have never seen it, but I know he worried. He worried about finances, and when he lost his job, he worried about finding a new one. He worried about me and he worried about his family as a whole. The feeling of loss of control also affected my dad. He was the fixer. If something broke, he could fix it. I was the one thing he could not fix. I cannot imagine how helpless he must have felt. My dad just wanted his normal life back; we all did.

I think my parents viewed my prognosis as an inconvenience, and that my cancer would eventually go away and I would get better. The goal was to get back to normal as soon as possible. Nothing prepared us for the next two and a half years. And I don't think we ever returned to normal.

A Funky Winkerbean comic said: "So tell me, Holly . . . After cancer do things ever return to normal?" "More or less . . . but eventually, you come to realize . . . normal isn't as normal as it once was."

Our normal changed. My family had to be flexible, and we soon learned life revolved around how I felt. On multiple occasions, we would be all set to drive to a family function, and I would get sick, forcing all of us or mom and me to stay home. Or we would have something planned and I would end up in the hospital with a fever. I never knew if I would wake up feeling well or if I would wake up feeling lousy. Our normal changed every day. I know it taught my dad to be flexible. As much as he likes routine, he knew my cancer wasn't routine. We used to have set plans, but now nothing was set; everything was day by day and sometimes moment by moment. Life was now divided by how we did things "before" my cancer and "after."

My diagnosis wasn't easy for my parents. I know it put a strain on their marriage. My dad didn't always agree with how my mom handled things and my mom didn't always agree with my dad. They experienced my diagnosis from two different viewpoints; my mom was in the trenches with me and my dad watched from the sidelines. I knew there was tension, although they did a good job at hiding it. I know Dad thought Mom did too much for me or didn't push me hard enough, but she wanted me to conserve my energy so I could enjoy myself when I was feeling well.

Mom struggled with balancing everything—caring for me, being the wife my dad needed, being a homemaker, and being a mom to my brother. When did she have time to take care of herself? I did my best to support her, to make her laugh. When you're on as high a dose of prednisone as I was, your whole body tends to swell. I had a huge belly and felt like the Pillsbury Doughboy. To make my mom laugh, I would poke myself in the belly and giggle like he did on the commercials.

Per the recommendations of my nurses and doctors, my parents attended a support group for parents of kids with cancer. The first two times they were glad they went because they received information on insurance and what to expect when you have a child with cancer. The third time, I was having a great day, the chemotherapy was working, and my parents wanted to share the good news, but before their turn came, others in the group were talking about the setbacks their children were having. When their turn came to share, they chose not to because they were the only ones who had good news to share. After that experience, they chose not to go back.

In retrospect, sharing my good news could have offered others hope, but they too were just learning how to navigate the world as parents of a child with cancer. They recognized the benefit of going, but in the end, discovered it wasn't for them.

Theresa was a freshman in college when I was diagnosed. When I asked her how she reacted, she told me she remembers thinking of me as a "weenie." She admits that was an immature response, but I think she knew she couldn't do anything, since she was so far away and was isolated from the entire situation. She was upset I was hogging all the attention. My sister couldn't understand why so many of her friends asked about me. Distance prevented her from seeing the reality of the situation.

Steven was a junior in high school at the time of my diagnosis. When I asked him years later how he felt, he said he was surprised and curious. I think he had it the hardest since he was still at home. His life changed because

Mom was at the hospital with me. Dad would come after work to visit me, and my brother was left to fend for himself. My parents tried to keep his life as normal as possible. Dad would walk to work so Mom could drive me to my clinic appointments, leaving Steven the second car so he could drive to school. I also think he felt forgotten. He had finally made academic honors, but he didn't know if our parents would notice because they were so busy with me. They did notice, but I was taking up most of their attention and time. I always felt guilty he didn't get the recognition he deserved for his achievement.

Neither my sister nor my brother understood the amount of pain I had been in during the previous months, and they would make fun of me because they thought I was being a wimp. After the diagnosis, they realized I had been in pain, and they didn't know how to act. They both felt I was hogging everyone's attention. Neither sibling visited me in the hospital much. My brother came on my birthday and later when I was in the PICU, but for the most part, he stayed away. I don't blame him. I just think he didn't know what to say, so he said nothing and that was OK.

I later found out through a friend of the family, Steven and his friends attempted to see me in the hospital, but there was a snowstorm that night, so they never made it. When I found out he tried, I smiled. My brother did care but just didn't know how to show it. He did go with me to a clinic appointment once and quickly found out how boring sitting in the clinic actually was. My sister came to the hospital once. She was home from college on break and came to see me while I was in isolation due to pneumonia. I don't blame her for never coming to see me; she lived two hours away and was enjoying her first year of college.

Everyone in my family had a different perspective on the situation. My mom saw everything because she was there taking care of me. My dad and my brother only saw me when I was at home. They saw some days I had energy and other days I didn't. They mostly saw the good stuff. They didn't see me getting the chemo, and they didn't see me get sick. What they saw was that I would go to the clinic and come home with gifts. At Children's Hospital, for every spinal tap or bone marrow biopsy, a child gets to pick a toy out of the toy box, and—you guessed it—I often came home with a stuffed animal. My sister saw nothing. She only knew what she was told by someone else.

I have come to understand siblings often feel left out. They often feel forgotten because life revolves around the sick child. Thankfully, there are now organizations that focus on siblings or the family as a whole. One example is A Kid Again in Ohio and Indiana. A Kid Again provides opportunities for families to do activities together so no one feels left out and they meet other families with similar stories.

My grandparents had different reactions. One set of grandparents showed me they were thinking of me through kind deeds and prayer. My grandma sent me a card every day, even though she was taking care of my grandpa. I loved those cards and looked forward to them each day. My grandpa kissed my picture every night on his way to bed. Due to distance and my grandfather's health, they were unable to visit me, so this was their way of showing me they cared and loved me. My grandpa and I also exchanged prayers. Every morning he would offer his day up for me, and in turn I would offer my day up for him. It was our way of supporting each other when neither of us was feeling well.

My other set of grandparents struggled to cope with

my diagnosis. I think my grandma took the news harder than I did. She couldn't understand how I could be excited to lose my hair and was appalled I had fun pulling it out. They called me on my fourteenth birthday when I was sleeping. My grandma misunderstood why I couldn't talk and instead of calling back, stopped calling altogether for almost a month. My dad ended up calling them to ask what they were doing. Why hadn't they called? Why hadn't they visited? He was upset and I was hurt.

I now realize they reacted that way because they didn't know how to react. They cried when they found out we had been granted A Special Wish because they thought it meant I was dying. We had to explain the wishes were not only for terminal patients but also for those with life-threatening diseases, and I was not going to die. When they did call, my grandma would always ask, "Are you up and running any races yet?" This was her way of asking how I was feeling.

I realized pets can be affected too. My parents adopted Misty for me when I was in the fifth grade. I had begged them for a dog for years, and they finally found one. Misty may have been adopted with the intention of being my dog, but she definitely was not my dog. She was my dad's dog. She followed him around, not me. Slept in his room, not mine. Misty changed when I started sleeping in the recliner and later when I came home from the hospital. For my entire treatment, she never left my side. She sat by my chair in the family room, slept next to my bed at night, and would only leave my side to go outside for a walk. She knew something wasn't right, and she was my comfort. Prior to my diagnosis, when I was sleeping in the recliner, Misty slept in the family room with me. Did she know I was sick before I did? When my treatment was over, Misty went back to being Dad's dog.

Cancer affects every family member differently. Each person has a different perspective. No perspective is wrong, but with this comes a need to understand and support one another. Cancer can either tear families apart or bring them together. Realizing cancer isn't just about the patient is the first step. Understanding everyone will cope differently is the second, and accepting everyone's viewpoint is third. These three steps are crucial to staying together as a family.

9

FRIENDSHIPS

*A*s with family relationships, cancer can either bring friends together or tear friendships apart. Cancer taught me a lot about friendships. It taught me I had unrealistic expectations of my friends. It taught me who my real friends were. It taught me you can find friends in the most unexpected places.

Cancer challenges friendships every step of the way. I found the people I expected to be by my side were the ones who disappeared. I didn't have the experience where everyone rallies around in support, no one shaved their head for me, and people weren't knocking down my door checking in on me. I think my classmates cared but just didn't know how to show it. Don't get me wrong, my classmates' parents set up a dinner calendar and people asked about me, but mostly it was the adults, not my peers.

The biggest obstacle to maintaining friendships with my classmates was the fact I had to drop out of school and get a tutor in order to keep up with my class and graduate on time. The plan was for me to return to school, but my parents didn't want me to miss too many days because of clinic appointments or not feeling well, and they were worried I would not be able to graduate on time. Having a tutor and not being part of a class isolated me from my classmates, who were able to move on with their lives while I was stuck trying to figure out my new life, which was now so very different from theirs.

One of my closest friends, Sam, was there for me when I was diagnosed. He and his parents were the first to visit me in the hospital. He brought me a stuffed dog. There was a bit of awkwardness during his visit: What do you say to someone who was just told they had cancer? Sam didn't know what to say and neither did I. But he came and that meant the world to me.

A couple of days later was my fourteenth birthday. My friends had arranged with my mom and the nurses to throw me a surprise birthday party. They came with a cake, which looked like a piece of cheese with a mouse in it. I had fun. I didn't have a lot of energy, but I did the best I could, and I loved being with my friends. I felt part of the group again.

Sadly, after my birthday many of them didn't come back to the hospital. A couple of classmates were given permission to miss school and spend the day with me in the clinic, but I felt horrible on those days and they ended up playing games while they sat with me. Looking back, I'm sure the classmates who did come learned a lot. They learned how boring clinic visits were and how sick chemo can make you. They also saw firsthand what I was going through. No one ever came back a second time, but years later one friend told me the experience helped him realize how strong I was for going through what I did.

The most common way to show support to someone who is sick is by sending them cards, a gift, flowers, praying for them, or making them dinner. People did all these things for me and I appreciated every one of them. However the one thing I needed most I didn't get: I needed company, I needed my friends. Why didn't people come? Why did my friends stop calling? Was it because their lives didn't stand still as mine did or because they didn't know what to say?

My math teacher thought it would be a good idea for my classmates to call me during her class. She had great intentions, but those phone calls felt forced, and many of the classmates who called were people I didn't normally hang out with. I appreciated the phone calls, but again, none of us knew what to say. I'm sure my classmates were concerned, and I will never know what they were thinking, but I do know being forced to call someone wasn't the answer.

My basketball team came over to my house after winning the championship game. My mom provided cake and ice cream and it felt good to be part of something again. It felt good to celebrate with my teammates even though I hadn't been at the game. But just like my birthday, everyone disappeared when it was over.

Nobody ever warned me of the side effects of cancer. I'm not talking about the physical effects, which I was lucky to avoid. I'm talking about the emotional and social effects—the loneliness. Two weeks after I was diagnosed, most of my friends weren't there for me. No one prepared me for that. Of course, it didn't help that they were told they could not visit me if they had a cough or a possible cold because they could give me an infection and I would not be able to heal as quickly as they did. It probably scared them. My illness was also something no one in my class had faced before. It wasn't a broken leg or the flu. This was different. I give them credit for sticking around for a few weeks, and I appreciated the few who came to clinic appointments with me, but eventually, it was just my mom and me. I was grateful for the time with my mom, but I missed being with friends.

Throughout my treatment, I had many delays, delays due to fevers and delays due to blood counts being too low. Sometimes it would take a week for my blood counts to get to the point they needed to be to continue chemotherapy. These delays pushed back my protocol phases. It just so happened that due to all the delays, I was between phases the last two weeks of my eighth-grade year. There was always a two- to three-week break between phases to rest the body. I typically felt good during those times since I didn't have chemo to take.

Because of the break, I was able to participate in some of the end of year fun. I got to go to the local water park with my eighth grade class for a class trip, but again I felt isolated. I was the only one who couldn't go swimming because I had a Broviac and couldn't get it wet, and no one wanted to miss out on swimming to hang out with me. They were able to be normal kids at a water park. I was just happy to feel good enough to be out of the house and around people.

Graduation night was a great night. There was a dance afterward and I got to celebrate with my class-mates. Everyone forgot about my cancer for one night, and we danced, had fun, and I got to be normal again. Sadly, as with my birthday, a few weeks after graduation I was alone again. This was the loneliest time for me. I don't recall talking to many friends that summer. Sam didn't call or visit much, although that was normal for us. We would go our separate ways during the summer and reconnect during the school year, but this summer was different. This summer I needed to feel normal. I needed to know that when I started high school in the fall, I would have friends. I was overjoyed when Sam called and asked if I wanted to go to freshman orientation together. It was nice hearing from him again. I had missed him. Our friendship picked up right where it had left off before I had cancer.

Three weeks into my freshman year, I was hospitalized for pneumonia. I had to stay in the hospital for three weeks. Two weeks in isolation and one week in the PICU. While I was there, many classmates came to visit me, many I hadn't even met yet. This was a hard time for Sam. He told me years later everyone always asked him where I was or how I was doing. I now understand the pressure he must have felt. People were always asking about me but not thinking about his feelings as well.

I think my diagnosis was the beginning of the end of my relationship with Sam. I think we tried, but in the end, I couldn't understand why he didn't get the "cancer" part of my life, and he didn't understand my need to cope with my cancer. Sam didn't get the support he needed from me, and I didn't get the support I needed from him. Deep down, I was jealous that he had a normal life and I didn't anymore. Our lives had changed, and we grew apart. One of the last things I remember him saying was that it was always about me. I cried when I heard him say that. I regret he felt that way, and I regret not being there for him. I will always love him and I wish we were still friends. In the end, if our friendship is meant to continue, it will, in time.

Cancer doesn't kill friendships, but a lack of understanding another person's needs does. Friendships can't be one-sided; you have to support one another. What I failed to do was understand where the other person was coming from. This lack of understanding went on to destroy more friendships. I was young and didn't have anyone to talk to about this. I did the best I could, but I learned some tough lessons along the way.

I was now a member of the cancer community. I didn't ask to be a member, but I was thrust into it the day I was diagnosed, and I was navigating being a survivor the best way I knew how. When I was surviving cancer, there weren't resources for what to do next. I had to figure it out on my own. I made mistakes. I put too much emphasis on understanding the "cancer" side of me. I expected everyone around me to understand me, but I didn't take the time to understand them. I expected people to support me. I judged friendships based on whether they would be there for me if I relapsed. I now know that was an unfair view of being a friend. I was so worried about people judging me for having cancer, that I didn't realize I was judging them.

I was diagnosed at a time when kids are figuring out who they are and finding independence from their parents. I didn't get to experience this because I was figuring out how to survive. I was going to a hospital three times a week, and I was dependent on my parents. I had a hard time connecting with my peers because I didn't experience this developmental stage. Due to everything I had been through, I felt I was emotionally older than my peers, but socially I felt younger. I could easily talk to people older than me and those younger than me, but I felt awkward with my peers, and it wasn't until my late twenties when everything worked itself out.

Missing the beginning of freshman year of high school was rough. The first month of freshman year is crucial to establishing new friendships. I missed out on building new friendships due to being hospitalized with pneumonia, and because of that I never felt I fit in. My grade school friends quickly made new friends, and I often felt I was just tagging along. I felt people were nice to me because they felt sorry for me. I was too focused on me and what I had been through to be a good friend to someone else.

I completed treatment in April of my sophomore year. I had only two years of high school where I felt like a normal teenager, as normal as it can be for someone who just beat cancer, but by then it was too late. I had no idea how to relate to my peers. I didn't know how to make new friends. I know my classmates tried to get to know me, and by the time I graduated I had friends, but not the lifelong kind. Not the kind I longed for.

I felt isolated from my classmates in other ways too. Sadly, in ways I could not control. I was bald. I loved being bald, but nothing sticks out more than a bald girl in a Catholic high school where everyone wears a uniform and looks the same. I was called "leukemia girl" and probably many other names. I had to leave school early for clinic appointments every week during my freshman and sophomore year. I couldn't participate in gym class, which wasn't necessarily a bad thing, but it was just one more thing that set me apart.

During gym class my sophomore year, I helped the teacher record the times my classmates were running the mile. I couldn't run or do anything physical, so helping her was at least one way I could be involved. The freshmen in my gym class didn't know anything about me; they didn't know I was going through cancer treatment. When everyone finished running and we were walking back to the locker rooms, I heard them talking about me, commenting on the fact I didn't run the mile like everyone else. I quickly turned around and told them I didn't run because I had cancer and was taking chemotherapy that prevented me from participating, and if they didn't want to run the mile, then they should get cancer, but I didn't recommend it. Needless to say, I didn't make any friends that day.

Cancer was part of my life, the only thing I knew. I spent two and a half years fighting it. I was just happy to be alive. I didn't play sports anymore; I wasn't a part of any clubs or other extracurricular activities. My priorities were different than those of my peers, and that had a tremendous effect on my relationships. For a long time, I wondered if my friends truly understood what I had to go through and how alone I felt. I felt I couldn't talk about my treatment with my friends. I felt the only people who really understood me were other cancer survivors because they had experienced it for themselves. Truth is, there is a side of me only those who have gone through cancer will get, but cancer doesn't define me, and there is a whole other side of me that people would see if I let them.

The problem was the wall I built to protect myself. The wall kept people out for fear of them hurting me, fear of them leaving me as so many had. It was my way of hurting someone first to prevent them hurting me. Many years later, two close friends convinced me that having a wall to protect myself was only hurting me. It prevented me from meeting people and prevented me from being a good friend.

My sophomore year I attended Heme Camp, a camp for kids with cancer. For the first time, I was surrounded by others like me. I loved it. I finally fit in and made some great friends. Sadly, this also had a way of isolating me from my "normal" friends. I remember during my senior year telling a friend I was excited to be able to return to camp. She responded, "Why do you want to go hang out with those people?" I immediately thought, does she consider me as one of "those" people? What did she mean by that? Needless to say, my friendship with her didn't last long, because at that time I judged friendships based on whether someone understood how important being a cancer survivor was to me.

Throughout college, I lost more friends to cancer. Not to the disease itself but to the lack of understanding why cancer was still at the forefront of my life. I constantly felt I was different. I viewed life differently and had different priorities. I figure that's what happens when you are given a second chance at life.

Once I had to take a friend to the emergency room. It was the same emergency room my dad took me to six years earlier. As I walked through the doors with my friend, I pictured my dad carrying me into the ER. I saw the exact spot where we sat to have my vitals taken and where my dad filled out paperwork. I thought back on that day when my life changed. When I got back to the dorm, I needed to talk with someone about my flashback because it was the first time I ever had one that intense. I told my friends about my flashback, and they said they didn't understand why it bothered me and why I felt I needed to share this with them. I was hurt, hurt they didn't want to listen to me, hurt they didn't understand my need to talk, and hurt they couldn't understand how cancer still could be affecting me years later. Again, another friendship ended because of my cancer.

Years later, I heard this quote from Lance Armstrong: "Cancer may leave your body, but it will never leave your life." I wish I'd heard this quote back in college. I would have understood why I needed to talk about my flashback, and I might not have lost friends over it. Looking back, I probably did talk about my cancer a lot. Probably too much. One thing I failed to realize is that not everyone wants to hear about it. For some, it brings up sadness, which was the case with a college roommate. Years later, when I reached out and asked what I did wrong, my room-mate told me that my talking about my survival reminded her that her mom didn't survive. To her, cancer meant death, not life. I knew her mom died of cancer, but I never considered how I must have made her feel.

I think overall, when someone experiences a major life-changing event, they have a need to talk about it much longer than people want to hear about it. It takes time to process life-changing events, and we need to understand, as the person experiencing the event, how others will feel listening to us. Our friends and family need to understand our need to process what just happened. I think by identi-fying that each person has needs, an overall understanding will take place.

Another time I got upset with a friend because he wouldn't go with me to my annual doctor's appointment at the Children's Hospital. He later told me that seeing sick children made him sad and he didn't want to cry in front of them. Seeing bald heads was normal for me, but I never considered what cancer or bald heads meant to others. We all come to the table with our own experiences of what cancer is. Knowing this helps.

Just as you have to meet a cancer patient where they are, to help them cope with a diagnosis, you also must approach friendships and any other relationship the same way. You can't expect someone to immediately understand and be there to support you. You have to also understand their history and what cancer means to them.

My cancer treatment was a lonely time for me. My greatest fear in life is being alone, but I have come to real-ize, you can be with a group of people and still feel alone. You can be alone without feeling lonely, and you can be happy when you're alone. I've also found that I am never truly alone. God is always with me.

SCHOOL

*B*eing diagnosed in the middle of my eighth-grade year wasn't easy. School was completely disrupted. I had the desire to finish school so I could stay on track with my friends, but I also had no desire to focus on school. My lack of focus started with the intense pain and continued as a side effect of the chemotherapy, but also that school just didn't seem that important to me; getting through each day was where my focus was.

To finish off the school year, my parents found a tutor for me. The interesting part was since I went to a private school, I couldn't get a tutor for free. My parents withdrew me from my school and enrolled me in the public school with the understanding I would continue to follow the private school curriculum. When the time came to graduate, I dropped out of the public school and re-enrolled in the private school so I could graduate with my class. Having a tutor was great. When I wasn't up to reading, she would read to me; when I didn't feel like writing, I would dictate to her and she would write my paper. She would give me my tests orally and I didn't have as much homework. My teachers knew I was busy trying to survive.

The transition to high school wasn't easy. The previous six months I had a tutor to help me with everything. Suddenly, I was thrust into having to do everything on my own again. I didn't have anyone to help me when I was tired. When I missed school because of the pneumonia, I fell even more behind. For the three weeks I had been in the hospital, I hadn't felt like working on homework. Most teachers understood and let me turn things in as I could. My history teacher was the most understanding. He told me to focus on all my other classes. He would give me an incomplete for the first quarter and would work with me after school the second quarter to get caught up. I'll never forget his patience and understanding.

The hardest part about surviving cancer was the expectation that I would return to a normal teenage life. How was I supposed to do that when I had never been a normal teenager? By the time I finished treatment I was sixteen, and the only teenage life I knew was hospitals and cancer treatment. How was I supposed to fit in when I nothing in common with my peers?

At the time, survivorship programs didn't exist to help me navigate life after cancer. I reached out to a childhood cancer group on the internet and I found a few friends online who had cancer. We helped each other figure life out, but none of us had any real advice to give because we were all experiencing it for the first time. After everything I had gone through, I struggled with my identity. My school friends were athletes or musicians. I couldn't play any sports anymore, I didn't have the energy to join clubs or extracurricular activities, and by the time I did, the clubs were already formed and friendships already created, and I didn't want to be the new member so late in the game. So, my identity became being a cancer survivor. I often feel I was cheated out of a true high school experience.

I felt people expected that once I completed my treatment I was just going to pick up where I left off and continue life. But life changes. Priorities change. Dreams change. Relationships change. It's not easy picking up the pieces and moving on. I discovered that life changes for everyone. My normal wasn't other people's normal, and that is OK. Because normal is different for everyone.

Over the years I have been jealous of people who I perceive to have "normal" lives. I was jealous of my siblings. For years, I wondered what they had to worry about. They don't worry about health insurance like I do. They don't worry about follow-up tests and secondary cancers. Their lives seem perfect, but then one day it hit me: It doesn't matter because no one's life is perfect. What is normal for one person might not be for another. A person's normal is an evolving feeling. A person's normal changes with a diagnosis, a marriage, a birth of a child, the death of a loved one, and so on.

I had always dreamt of working with animals, so after high school I attended The Ohio State University to study zoology. There, my identity crisis continued, but the difference was no one knew my history. All my high school classmates knew I had cancer, knew I had to leave class to go to the hospital, knew I couldn't do everything they did because I was regaining my strength and rebuilding my immune system. But my college friends had no idea. They all talked about everything they had done in high school, what sports they played, the art they had created, the people they dated. I didn't do any of those things. All I did was beat cancer. Cancer was all I knew so that's what I talked about. I later came to find out my friends thought I talked about my cancer too much, which made some of them uncomfortable.

I couldn't relate to my classmates in high school because I didn't have the energy to do the things they did, and I couldn't relate to my college friends because I didn't do anything in high school and had nothing to talk about. No one wanted to hear about what I did pre-cancer in middle school; they didn't care I was the best bunter in softball in the seventh grade.

While in college, my doctors wanted me to be tested for any learning disabilities, due to the cranial radiation I had received. On the day of my appointment, I had to leave organic chemistry early. I told my professor at the beginning of class I had a doctor appointment and needed to leave early. As I got up to leave, he jokingly asked if a doctor's appointment was more important than organic chemistry. I replied that going to see the doctor to see if I had a learning disability caused by radiation from cancer treatment is. The look on my professor's face was priceless. I guarantee he wasn't expecting that for my answer. The test revealed no learning disabilities, but my professor didn't need to know that, he pulled me aside the next class and offered to allow me to take my tests in his office with no time limit. Since I struggled with organic chemistry, I played the cancer card and took him up on his offer.

In my final quarter at OSU, I completed an internship at the Dolphin Research Center in the Florida Keys. It was there that realized I could combine my love of animals with my desire to help others. When my internship was over, I decided to pursue a master's degree in recreational therapy. Being a recreational therapist would allow me to do what I love. Animal-assisted therapy was a common intervention used in this profession and I knew I might be able to work with pediatric cancer patients one day. I had always known I wanted to give back, and being a recreational therapist was a way I could. I earned my child life specialist certification while working at a children's hospital.

After college graduation, I continued to meet people who didn't know I had cancer. I wondered at what point in a relationship I should tell someone I had leukemia. Some people choose to never disclose it, but I felt if people didn't know I had cancer, they couldn't know me. It played such an important part of my life and it was the reason I did the things I did and believed what I believed.

I didn't date in high school and I didn't date in college. I think I didn't date because I was trying to figure out who I was. I was twenty-three years old when I met my first boyfriend. Shortly after I met him, we were walking in a park getting to know each other. We were talking about our lives when it came up that he had gone to the emergency room when he had his fingers slammed in a car door. A nurse had to stick a needle into the tip of his finger. He said there was no pain greater than that. I quickly replied I'd had cancer and there was no greater pain than what I had gone through. My boyfriend was shocked, and we laughed since he agreed his finger pain didn't compare to my back pain. I learned at some point in every relationship an opportunity to tell someone about what I went through will present itself and I didn't need to force the conversation. I realized then I didn't need to be so serious. I could have fun with my story. I did enjoy one-upping him that day.

Another time the subject just naturally flowed into the conversation was at a friend's party. Someone mentioned they had to have ACL surgery at sixteen and how painful that was. My friend replied, "I had a baby at fifteen." I quickly replied, "I had cancer at fourteen." My friend turned to me and laughingly said, "No one has ever beaten me at this before."

I have learned not every person in my life needs to know I had cancer. I used to think cancer defined me. It doesn't. Our pasts do not define us, but they do influence our actions and thoughts in a positive or negative way. I use my past as inspiration to get involved and make a difference. To ensure future kids with cancer don't have to go through what I went through. To ensure they don't go through it alone.

Live Life, Love Life, Cherish Every Moment

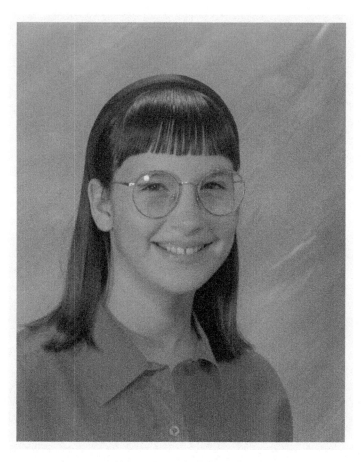

October 1993 - 8th Grade School Picture

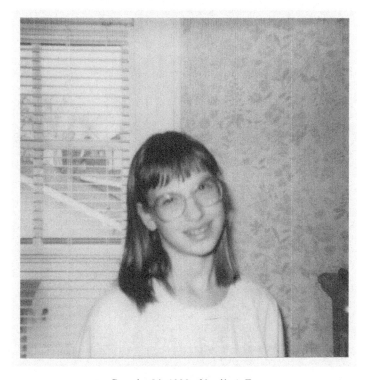

December 31, 1993 - New Year's Eve

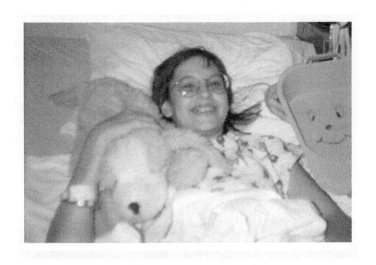

January 1994 - Me and my stuffed dog, Katie

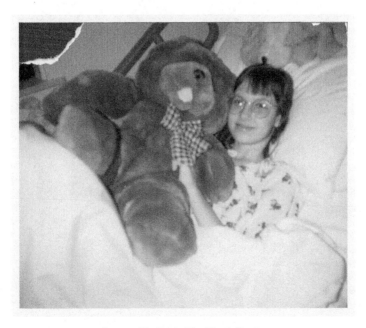

January 30, 1994 - First Hospitalization

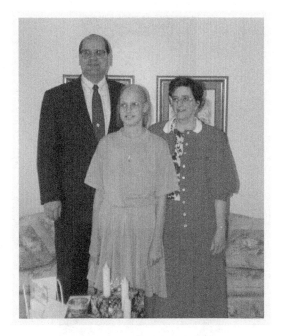

May 1994 - My Parents and I

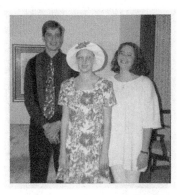

June 1994 - 8th Grade Graduation

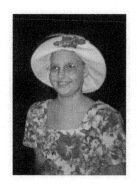

August 1994

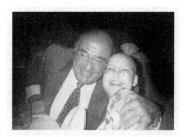

August 1994 - Uncle John and I

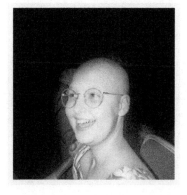

August 1994

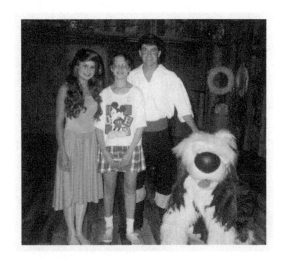

June 1995 - Special Wish Trip

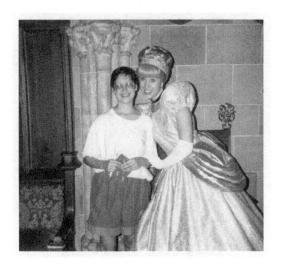

June 1995 - Special Wish Trip

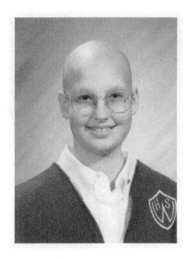

September 1994 - Freshman Year

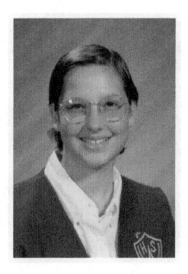

September 1995 - Sophomore Year

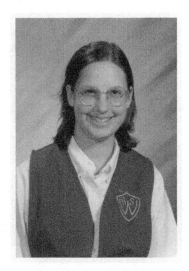

September 1996 - Junior Year

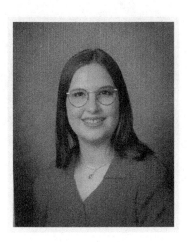

August 1997 - Senior Year

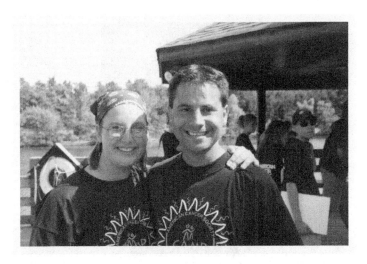

August 1999 - Camp Friendship

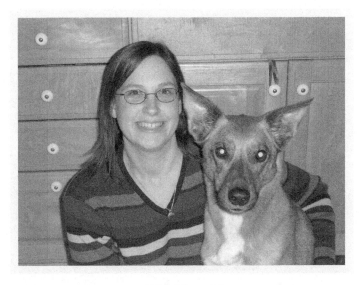

2004 - Velvet and I

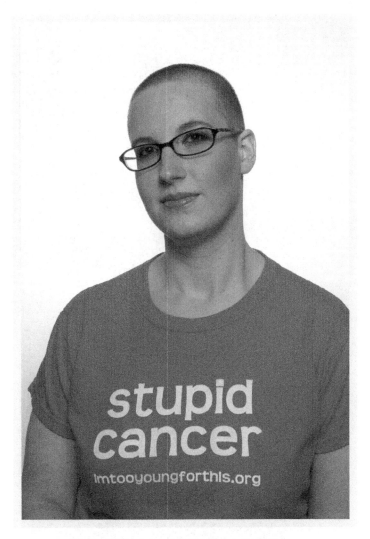

February 2009 - Bald is Beautiful, Photo by Mark Jackman

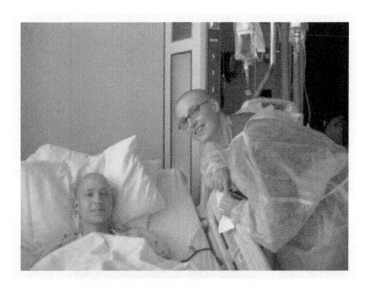

March 2009 - Working as a Recreational Therapist

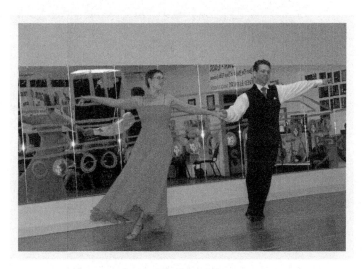

2011 - Ballroom Dancing with Daniel, Photo by Steve Miller

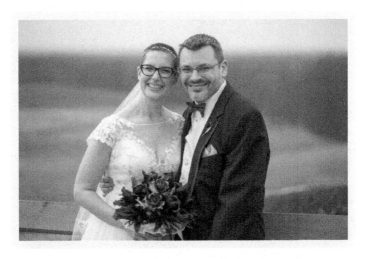

March 2017 - Wedding Day, Photo by Black Dog Photo Co.

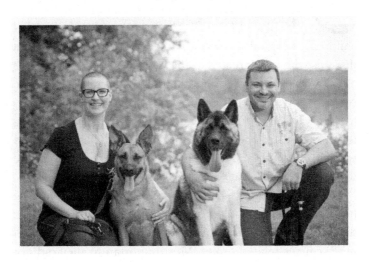

July 2017 - My Family, Photo by Black Dog Photo Co.

THE HAPPIEST PLACES ON EARTH

*H*eme Camp (Hematology Camp) was the first place I felt as if I fit in. It was run by the local children's hospital for those with cancer or blood-related diseases who were treated at the hospital. Heme Camp was a place where I forgot about the real world and lived in the moment. I was free to be me and was surrounded by others like me. I found out about the camp shortly after being diagnosed but didn't attend for another two years until I was off chemotherapy. I feared the chemo would interfere with having fun. That was a decision I would later regret.

During my first year at camp, I met people outside the hospital environment who were my age, with my same diagnosis, who knew about Broviacs and prednisone and other cancer-related topics. Most importantly, they did not treat me differently because I had cancer. Camp took my isolation away and allowed me to make lifelong friendships. I met campers who lived near me. It was great having friends close by, friends whom I would never have met if it had not been for camp and cancer.

After camp we didn't want the fun to end, so we convinced our parents to take us to a nearby restaurant so we could continue talking. Our parents didn't mind, they enjoyed talking with each other. We would talk for hours about camp, our cancers, and being sick. We always laughed that by the time we left, none of the tables around us had any people sitting there. We would joke that we scared them off by our cancer conversations. This tradition continued year after year. When I became too old to be a camper, I transitioned into being a counselor, as did many others.

Heme Camp was run from the heart. The dedicated counselors, nurses, and doctors who volunteered their time at camp each year proved this. We were a dedicated and passionate group of individuals who came from all walks of life. There were many counselors who had been coming to camp for over ten years, and some who drove from other states or flew from other countries to volunteer at Heme Camp. My fellow counselors and I returned year after year for the children, our own memories of camp motivating us.

This camp was not like other camps. Heme Camp was not just a summer camp for kids. It was a place where kids who are picked last at school are picked first, where kids who sit alone at lunch at school because they are different sit among friends. Camp provided a safe place where life-long friendships with unique bonds were built. One camper stated, "We share a bond of our sickness." Camp was a place where we forgot the real world. It was a place where everyone, campers and staff, was included and no one felt like an outsider. I looked forward to going back each year and seeing each camper grow and thrive as a survivor.

One of my fondest memories at Heme Camp was

water balloon battleship. The campers would be on the edge of the lake with hundreds of water balloons and slingshots, while the counselors would get in canoes, kayaks, and pedal boats. The campers would then take aim at the counselors in the boats. By the end of the activity, everyone was soaking wet. Campers had a great time launching balloons at their counselors and the counselors had fun throwing the balloons back at their campers and tipping other counselors' boats. The best part was when new counselors would get in the pedal boats thinking they were safe. What they didn't know was with enough effort, those tip too.

Heme camp always ended with a dance on the last night. The first song played was always "Celebration" by Kool & the Gang and the dance always ended with everyone holding hands in a circle, singing and crying to "That's What Friends Are For" by Dionne Warwick. To many, Disney World is the happiest place on Earth, but for me Heme Camp was. It was a place where you lived in the moment, you laughed, you cried, and you were among friends.

Another camp I was a part of for a few years was Camp Friendship through the American Cancer Society. I found out about the camp in my English 101 class during my freshman year at The Ohio State University. We were proofreading other students' essays and I was proofreading one on Camp Friendship and another student was reading mine about being a cancer survivor. The next year I joined her at camp.

One benefit of having cancer as a child is you always have a topic for any paper needed at school. I think I was able to write about cancer for most of my high school and college papers. This is an excerpt of one paper I wrote in college, written July 14, 1999.

What Camp Friendship meant to me . . .

Camp Friendship means more to me than one would think. It gave me a chance to meet new people and make new friends. It also gave me the ability to accomplish things I hadn't done since I got sick. True, it's been five years since I was sick, but there are many things I haven't done since then. I was able to play sports again. I was able to run and be free without a care in the world. I hadn't played basketball, softball, or volleyball since I was sick. I was so proud of myself that I did all those things. To anyone else, those sports may be something so easy and some might laugh when I said I was proud of myself, but it meant the world to be able to play again.

Camp Friendship is a place where we are ourselves and do not have to hide the fact we had cancer. We accept everyone for who they are, even if they are missing a leg or an arm or a shoulder. No matter what, you are a part of our cancer survivor community. At camp we share our experiences with each other, we talk about those who have died, and most importantly, we have fun being normal.

At both Heme Camp and Camp Friendship, we had many inside jokes. Outsiders might see our jokes as sick and twisted, but for us they were a part of camp. No one was offended because we all knew everyone was joking around. First-year campers were often afraid to join in, but after they saw how much fun we had by joking about our cancer, they quickly joined in.

One of my favorite things about Camp Friendship was how we chose teams, which was based on what kind of cancer you had. It began when we were talking about how leukemia is the most common type of childhood cancer and Ewing's sarcoma is supposedly the least common. However, at camp, there were almost as many kids with Ewing's sarcoma as there were with leukemia. We found this funny and decided to see who was better, kids with leukemia or Ewing's. When it was time to play a game, blood cancers (leukemia) were on one team and bone cancers (sarcoma) were on the other. People who wanted to play but had a rare form of cancer were then picked one by one to even out the teams.

Another comment we often used when we did not want to participate was: "I can't do that; didn't you know I have cancer." Everyone knew you had cancer because it's a camp for kids with cancer, and you wouldn't be at camp if you did not have it, but we all said it because we thought it was funny. In the outside world, you can use the cancer card to get out of doing something or to get something you want, but using the cancer card here didn't work. You can't use the cancer card on other cancer survivors.

My favorite memory isn't a very nice one. We were at camp the same time as another group of campers. The campground was large enough to accommodate two small camps. The other camp was a "just say no to drugs" camp. Our head counselors thought it would be a good idea to have a shared camp dance. Well, good in theory but not in reality. The other campers treated us like we had the plague. We just wanted to have fun and they wouldn't dance and barely talked to us. The next day we decided to have a little fun. We took sidewalk chalk and wrote "drugs saved our lives," "I take drugs," and our nurse wrote, "I'm a drug dealer." In reality, chemotherapy is the harshest form of drug there is, so yes, drugs did save our lives and our nurse ensured those of us currently in treatment got our chemo, so in theory, he was a drug dealer. We wrote those things just to have a little fun, but it angered the other campers, so we were forced to wash the chalk off the sidewalk. But our fun didn't end there. I mentioned before that many cancer survivors have a twisted sense of humor. Well, we decided to spread a rumor: mosquitoes can spread leukemia. To someone who doesn't know much about cancer, it sounds plausible. Leukemia is a blood cancer and mosquitoes suck our blood and go from person to person feeding. I'm not sure if the other campers believed it, but we sure had a good laugh.

Both Heme Camp and Camp Friendship meant so much to me. I looked forward to camp just as much as I looked forward to my birthday or Christmas. Camp was where I felt I belonged, a place where I was like everyone else. As I got older, I made sure I got the time off from work and planned my vacation days around it to ensure I'd be able to go.

Camps weren't the only happy places. I first heard about Adventures for Wish Kids (AFWK), now known as A Kid Again, while I was sitting in the waiting room at Children's Hospital in 1997. I was waiting for them to call my name so I could have my blood drawn when I heard kids talking about AFWK and an upcoming trip to Kings Island theme park. They were talking enthusiastically about it and it piqued my curiosity. They told me Adventures for Wish Kids was an organization that sponsored many events throughout the year for kids "like us" and the next "adventure" was going to be at Kings Island, the local amusement park. When we got home from the clinic, my mom called AFWK and signed us up.

The best part was it included the entire family. My first

"adventure" was going to Kings Island, and it left an impression on me. Imagine the surprise when my brother and sister were each given $20.00 to spend at the park. They finally felt it was cool to have a sister with cancer. We got a picnic lunch and admission to the park. It was a great family day. A few months later, we attended a Christmas party and once again, my siblings were included, and they too received a gift.

AWFK is a volunteer-run organization and I saw how many people care about kids like me, who often feel left out of the fun because of their illness. When I became too old to be an Adventure Kid, I became a volunteer. Adventures for Wish Kids allows kids with life-threatening illnesses to have fun with their family year-round. It is a place of hope, a place to forget the real world and be a kid. Years later, the organization changed its name to A Kid Again, because that is truly what it did, allowed kids to be a kid again.

A Special Wish Foundation was the wish-granting organization where I lived. At first, I wasn't going to make a wish. I wasn't as sick as some of the other children we had met, and even though I had been through a lot, I figured Special Wish needed to spend their resources on those kids, not me. My mentor Kelly convinced me to go. She explained the Special Wish Foundation *wants* to grant wishes to kids like me and it was a once-in-a-lifetime opportunity. When you are given an opportunity to wish for anything you want, the possibilities are endless. I thought about meeting someone, but there wasn't anyone famous I wanted to meet, so I decided to go on a trip so my whole family could be involved. My brother and sister were in college and I knew this would be the last family vacation we took. I chose to go to Disney World, which turned out to be the most popular wish.

The summer after my freshman year of high school I went on my Special Wish trip. The longest limousine I had ever seen picked us up at our house and drove us to the airport. We flew to Florida and were provided with a rental car. We drove to the Give Kids the World (GKTW) Village, which is a magical place in its own right. The village is where families stay during their Wish Trip to Disney World. At the village you are greeted by volunteers and given your own private villa. They do their best at making the Wish Kid feel special. The staff and volunteers provide so many special treats for the Wish Kids and their families. I won't go into details here because I don't want to ruin the special surprises for future wish families. Once you are part of the GKTW family, you are always a part of their family, and I enjoy going back to visit when I am in Florida.

Disney World goes above and beyond for their Wish Kids. I was given a special button that was my pass to the front of the line—think of it as the ultimate fast pass. My brother and sister thought the whole idea of the Give Kids the World Village and going to Disney World was childish, until they realized the power this special button had. We went to Magic Kingdom, Epcot, MGM, and Universal Studios. We ate at Hard Rock Café, pet baby alligators at Gatorland, and had a knight's feast at King Henry's Feast. Everywhere I went, people went out of their way to ensure I was having the best time ever. When I was too hot and needed to take a break, Disney cast members escorted us to the VIP lounges, which I didn't know existed.

I bought an autograph book and decided to have various characters sign it. I have a few special memories of autographs. The first was at the Indiana Jones stunt show. After the show, I asked a crew member if I could meet Indiana Jones for his autograph and picture. He had already left the set to shower, but when he was told there was a Wish Kid, he got dressed again and came out to meet me and sign my autograph book. I was also allowed to stay after the Little Mermaid show to get the autographs of Ariel and Prince Eric. Max the dog came out to see me too and I was able to have my picture taken with all of them. Under normal circumstances, this wouldn't have been possible, but because I was a Wish Kid, they made it happen.

Another memory at Universal Studios was at the animal actors show. Lassie appeared in the show, and since I grew up watching *Lassie* reruns, I asked for Lassie's autograph. I'm sure you're wondering how Lassie was going to sign my autograph book. It was easy: her trainer had Lassie bite my book. I know it wasn't the real Lassie, but I enjoy looking at my autograph book and seeing Lassie's bite mark.

My favorite and most special memory was with Cinderella. It was the hottest day we were there, and my family was outside watching a parade. It was too hot for me, so I was sitting inside Cinderella's castle when I saw Cinderella. Everyone was outside, so I got to visit with Cinderella for twenty minutes all by myself. She asked if there were any characters I was missing an autograph from. I told her Donald Duck and Sleeping Beauty. She took my book, went upstairs, and a few minutes later came back with Donald Duck's signature. As for Sleeping Beauty, she asked me for my address. A week later, I received an autographed picture of Sleeping Beauty standing in front of her castle in Disneyland. Cinderella didn't have to do those things for me, but by doing so she gave me memories that will last a lifetime. I left Florida with 163 autographs. When my trip was over, once again we were picked up at the airport by a stretch limousine and driven home.

I highly recommend that anyone who qualifies for a

Special Wish or Make-a-Wish takes it. It doesn't matter what you wish for, you and your family will build a lifetime of memories. Also, get involved with local organizations. They want to help, and you will meet people who understand what you are going through and make lifelong friends.

DOLPHINS

*L*earning about the healing power of dolphins started when I was in the hospital. Some nurses and doctors joked that one of the side effects I had from chemotherapy was laughter. I was able to see the positive in everything and was constantly giggling. I earned the nickname Pollyanna because of this. One day Mom and I were laughing while I was getting my chemo, and one of my doctors happened to walk by. He said laughter is the best medicine because each time you laugh, your body releases endorphins, which help the body heal. Mom and I shortened endorphins to "dolphins," because it was a lot easier and just more fun to say and I believed dolphins truly do have a healing power.

During those early days, my mom would give me "dolphins" to cheer me up, and occasionally when I saw her getting tired, I would give her one or two. Over the years, I have shared the need for "dolphins" with other newly diagnosed friends in the hope they will find a way to create their own healing endorphins.

Dolphins are my symbol of hope and survival. I have a

necklace with two charms, one with two dolphins and another with a dolphin's fluke. The two dolphins—one silver and one gold represent the two lives I have lived, one before cancer and the one I live now after cancer. I am a forever-changed person because of my experience. The dolphin fluke reminds me of the time I spent working with dolphins and how special they are. It's a replica of Pandora's tail, the dolphin I felt the strongest connection with.

During my senior year of college, I was an intern at the Dolphin Research Center (DRC) in the Florida Keys. It was there I realized I really did have a connection with a dolphin. My supervisor told me a story of how Pandora, a five-year-old dolphin, picked me. When my supervisor was deciding on interns, she would go down to the lagoons and show the dolphins the applications. On that day, Pandora was the only dolphin interested in the applications. My supervisor flipped through each page so Pandora could look at them. Pandora looked at all of them and then touched mine. Pandora picked me! My first interaction with her, and I wasn't even there. When I got to DRC, Pandora was first dolphin to interact with me. She tossed seaweed at me, in hopes I would toss it back and play with her.

One day during my internship, a young girl came to swim with the dolphins through the Make-A-Wish Foundation. She had a form of cancer with a 15 percent survival rate. She and other patients in Europe were on experimental drugs, and of the fifteen who started the treatment, only four were still alive. Her best friend had died the week before of the same cancer she had. This four-year-old decided she did not want to continue treatment; she figured she was going to die either way. Her doctors told her and her family to get out of the country and go do something fun and motivational to get her mind off treatment and cancer. They came to DRC. While they were there, the father dropped his camera in the water and ruined it. Knowing what an important day this was going to be, I bought him two disposable cameras from the gift shop. He was incredibly happy and grateful to be able to capture these moments.

During the girl's swim, she laughed and giggled, and you could tell she was having a wonderful time. She swam with A.J. and Pax, and she and her mom got to do so many activities with them: throw rings and balls, bob up and down (her favorite), and many others. After the swim, she got to pet Loki the sea lion and feed Kilo, another sea lion, an ice cube through the fence. At the end of the week, the little girl told her mom she wanted to go back to the hospital and start treatment so she could come back the following year. The motivation worked. Before they left, I told her parents I was a cancer survivor and gave them a poem of "What Cancer Cannot Do." The father became tearful, as did I, and the mother was so grateful to be able to talk to someone who understood and someone who could offer them hope.

When I found out this family was coming, I was unsure how a day with the dolphins could motivate a little girl to go back into the hospital. I knew why the family was coming, and I knew firsthand how this child felt. I, too, had experienced the loss of will to continue treatment when two friends died of the same thing I had. Why continue when you're going to die anyway? However, God took care of things. His plan was for Pax and A.J. to convince her to go back. During the three months I was at DRC, I saw many smiles because of the dolphins, but nothing as touching and as magical as that day. The dolphins gave her hope. The dolphins gave her "dolphins."

Dolphins are good at giving people "dolphins" by just

being themselves. You can't help but laugh or smile when you watch their silly antics. Remember to laugh, releasing your "dolphins" every day. Some days will be better than others, but always remember the healing power of dolphins.

What Cancer Cannot Do

Cancer is so limited …
It cannot cripple love
It cannot shatter hope
It cannot corrode faith
It cannot destroy peace
It cannot kill friendships
It cannot suppress memories
It cannot silence courage
It cannot invade the soul
It cannot steal eternal life
It cannot conquer the spirit

— AUTHOR
UNKNOWN

13

BALD IS BEAUTIFUL

*F*or many, the point in which cancer becomes real is when you start to lose your hair. A bald head is synonymous with having cancer. It's like a calling card telling the world you are sick. For me, having my hair fall out was one perk of having cancer. The thought of losing my hair never bothered me. At the time of my diagnosis, my dark brown hair was shoulder length. Since we knew it was going to fall out, Mom called our beautician, Patti, to come and cut my hair to a more manageable length, to make it easier when I began to lose it. It was emotional for her, she had known me since I was three years old, and it was hard for Patti to think of me being so sick.

As I slowly started to lose my hair, I would wake up with strands on my pillow. It wasn't until March I noticed large clumps of hair coming out. I was watching TV when I pulled the first handful of hair out. It's the oddest sensation in the world to pull out clumps of hair without it hurting. That day I pulled my hair out one handful at a time, until only wisps were left. These eventually fell out too. This was something I truly enjoyed doing; as I said before, I didn't like my hair and I didn't mind losing it. On occasion, during the breaks between phases, my hair would start to grow back but would quickly fall out again once I restarted chemo.

As part of our eighth-grade graduation tradition, each member of the class had a silhouette made. I was too sick to go to school to have mine done, so the mother in charge came to our house. I had no hair at the time, so she graciously added hair to the silhouette so I could look like I did prior to getting sick. On graduation day, I was between treatments and could take part in the ceremony with my class. I remember getting ready for graduation practice during the day and kidding around with my classmates saying, "I wonder how I'll style my hair tonight." I had found the perfect hat to match my graduation dress—a "Blossom" hat. *Blossom* was a show on TV in the mid-nineties and the main character, Blossom, wore hats with big flowers on them. Blossom hats were very popular at the time and I think maybe the only time I ever wore flowers in my life.

When the doctors told me I was going to lose my hair, they recommended getting a "hair prosthesis." At the time, if you called it a wig, the insurance company would not pay for it. I went to a wig salon and tried on a few. None of the wigs were styled the way I wore my hair. Most of the wigs were styled for old ladies, not a teenager, but they did their best to find one for me. I ended up getting one a little darker than my natural color, but the wig was so much thicker than my natural hair, I never felt comfortable wearing it. Plus, it was hot and itchy. I stuck my wig under the bathroom sink and there it stayed. I still have it and occasionally put it on for fun or wear it as part of a Halloween costume. One Halloween when I put it on, my dog barked at me. My own dog didn't even recognize me with the wig on.

It was a custom at Children's Hospital to give girls baseball caps with ponytails sticking out of the back. Cute idea, but again, I did not want to wear a baseball cap with or without a ponytail. When you have no hair, the plastic piece in the back of a baseball cap hurts, so my advice to anyone thinking of giving a hat to someone who has cancer is to find one without the plastic adjustable part on the back. The softer the better when it comes to a bald head. My favorite thing to wear was a do-rag, a blue bandana. I wore it most places, more to please everyone else since, I was perfectly fine being bald. I was often told I looked good bald because I had a nicely shaped head. It was an odd compliment, but one I enjoyed nonetheless.

My grandparents thought I should always wear a hat, but it wasn't me, and I liked who I was without my hair and without a hat. I was just happy to be able to go places and not feel sick. At my cousin's wedding, I wore my graduation dress with matching hat. I was sitting with my Uncle John who was bald and thought it would be fun to take off my hat and take a picture of our bald heads. Everyone gasped. That was the moment I realized everyone else cared more about me losing my hair than I did.

One day I did wear a baseball hat to church, and I had my first run-in with prejudice. It was taken off my head by another churchgoer during Mass and was told boys do not wear hats in church. I was so taken aback by what she did, I quickly put my hat back on. I had every right to wear my hat in church. Throughout the Mass, this individual continued to whisper about boys not wearing hats in church. I thought to myself, how religious she must be to be more focused on me than on the priest. I never had a chance to correct her. I didn't feel the need to disrupt Mass to tell her my situation, and when Mass was over, she disappeared too quickly for me to say something. I guess prejudice and preconceived ideas are everywhere.

Oddly enough, I saw more prejudice in church than anywhere else. Our church was having an Anointing of the Sick day and had reserved rows in the front for people who were sick. I was still going through treatment and had what would be considered a boy haircut at the time. My dad and I sat down in the reserved row. I felt the lady behind me tap me on the shoulder. When I turned around, she told me I was sitting in the row for people who were sick, and I needed to move. My dad, being the protector he is, quickly turned around and told the lady I had cancer and was there to get anointed. The look of shock on her face and the joy on mine as I smiled at my dad was great! I never let the prejudice I saw in church stop me from going to Mass. It just made me realize we all have a different perspective and relationship with God and sadly, oftentimes the most religious can also be the most judgmental.

Being bald as a freshman in high school made me stand out, but gradually my hair began to grow back, although it didn't change much and was still very thin. I was told many times my hair could grow back curly, thicker, or even a different color, but it didn't. I got the same stick-straight, thin, impossible-to-style hair. I love my high school pictures, which show the progression of my hair growth. I find the pictures amusing and enjoy looking back on how different I looked. It wasn't until many years later that I accepted the fact I wasn't meant to have hair. I was not given good hair at birth and I wasn't blessed with good hair the second time around either. In my opinion, God didn't intend for me to have hair.

I lost my hair for good when I heard about a head-shaving event sponsored by the St. Baldrick's Foundation. St. Baldrick's is the number-one organization funding childhood cancer research and raising awareness about childhood cancer. At the time there were not many girls or women who got their head shaved. Most of the participants were men, like the local fire department or fathers of patients. Local barbers and beauticians donated their time to do the head shaving. I decided I wanted to take part and my parents came to the event to support me. One of the volunteer beauticians happened to be the mother of one of my patients. When it came time for me to get my head shaved, she was the one to do it. While she was shaving my head, another beautician leaned over and whispered in my ear, "You have a beautifully shaped head." I laughed, remembering how many times I had been told that fifteen years earlier.

When I told a friend of mine who was a photographer what I was doing, he argued that a woman can't be beautiful bald. I told him I disagreed, and as a result of our disagreement, a week after I shaved my head, he took glamor shots of me. We were both amazed at how they turned out. I decided bald is beautiful. Confidence for me is a shaved head. After the photo shoot, I went home and wrote this:

How shaving my head changed my life.

Back in January 1994, when I was told I had leukemia, I immediately asked my doctor if I was going to lose my hair. When he told me I would, I was thrilled. I had always hated my hair; it was much too thin, straight, and I couldn't do anything with it. I loved being bald. It was fun pulling my hair out; it's the weirdest feeling when you can pull hair out without feeling it. I remember being told by many people that I had a nicely shaped head. It's a strange compliment, but a great one to hear, especially when you have no hair.

Jumping forward to January 2009, I decided to shave my head for St. Baldrick's in February. I always knew one day I would shave my head and St. Baldrick's provided me with an opportunity to do so. When I told people what I was doing, most reactions were "it will be so freeing and empowering." I laughed at their comments and thought "That's not why I'm doing this. How is it going to be freeing and empowering? I'm shaving because I loved being bald; I'm raising money for pediatric cancer research." Plus, I figured my hair would only take a year to grow back to the length it was.

February 28th was the day. That morning while I was in the shower I remember thinking "goodbye hair, goodbye conditioner" and when I was finished styling my hair I put my brush and blow dryer under the sink, knowing I would not be using them for many months. I was excited the whole day, and finally, it was my turn to go on stage to have my head shaved. I remember being slightly nervous because I didn't know what I would look like and if I would still have a nicely shaped head. As my head was getting shaved, it tickled, and I could feel the cold air on my scalp with each pass of the razor. It was one of the coldest days of the year and we were in an outside tent. As I sat in the chair getting shaved, one of the hairdressers who volunteered to shave heads leaned over to tell me I have a nicely shaped head. I laughed because she didn't realize I had been told that many times fifteen years earlier.

When I left the stage with my shaved head, everyone told me I looked great. Even people who didn't know me said how beautiful I was, and how I could pull off the "shaved head" look. I was amazed since I had never considered myself a beautiful girl. When I finally looked in the mirror, I hardly recognized myself. I was not prepared for the change that would take place within me over the next few days. Before, when I had hair, when I looked in the mirror, I would see a pretty person but never used the word "beautiful" to describe myself. I now believe in some ways my hair held me back. Even after cancer treatment when my hair grew back, it was thin. I never knew how to style it, never knew how to make it look good, and in some ways, my hair made me self-conscious. With a shaved head, I don't have to worry if a hair is out of place or starting to look stringy, which thin hair usually does after a few hours. Now, when I look in the mirror, I am amazed at how beautiful I feel and I smile.

Shaving my head has been one of the greatest decisions I ever made. I now know what everyone meant when they said shaving my head would be freeing and empowering. With this newfound confidence, I started to embrace my femininity. This was a shock to my family since they all knew me as the girl in the comfortable clothes, who hated to be called "cute," never wore makeup, and would only wear "girly" clothes if I was forced to. I have since bought makeup *and* use it daily, bought "girly" clothes *and* enjoy wearing them, and have decided to make sure I look "cute" even when I run errands or go hang out at the dog park. I had professional pictures taken, and again I was amazed at how beautiful they were. I feel the beauty I always felt was within me is now shown on the outside as well.

Bald is Beautiful!

A year later, I let my hair grow. I had promised one of my

patients he could shave my head at the St. Baldrick event his family was hosting. He was so excited. He did a good job, and the beauticians helped. The second time around, people asked why I did it again. Most people thought it was a one-and-done deal and I would let my hair grow back because that is what people did. So, I wrote another essay to share why I did it a second time.

Why I do it.

Unfortunately, there is a stigma that goes along with being a bald woman. It's not socially appropriate. Older women look at me without saying a word. Children look at me with "ahh" and a smile on their face, often commenting to their mothers that I have no hair. Then there are the women who come up to me and tell me their hair used to look like mine while they were going through cancer treatment. I congratulate them on being a survivor and explain I too am a survivor, but voluntarily shave my head to raise money and awareness for childhood cancers. They are usually amazed I would want to be bald again.

As I have discovered, some people wonder why I continue to shave my head for St. Baldrick's. I usually tell people it's because I am a sixteen-year childhood cancer survivor and I have lost too many friends to cancer and I want it to stop. But I want to let everyone in on a little secret: Shaving my head also makes me happy. Believe it or not, I enjoy being bald, and I love the St. Baldrick's Foundation. They give me a reason to shave my head. Being bald gives me a freedom I didn't ever feel when I had hair. It gives me the confidence to go out and conquer the world. It gives me a sense of being alive and living in the moment. I love the way my head feels. Being bald also allows me to continue to raise awareness about cancer and be an example to other cancer survivors that bald is beautiful.

In the end, I do it because of how it makes me feel on the inside. If I inspire other women to shave their heads, or I empower another woman to have the confidence to embrace her baldness during cancer treatment, that is just icing on the cake for me.

There was only one time I decided to try to grow my hair out to my original length. Oddly enough, it was when I met my husband. Looking back on those pictures, I don't know what I was thinking or more importantly what *he* was thinking, especially since he said he was a "hair guy" and I definitely didn't have pretty hair. A month after meeting him, I shaved my head. I am happy to report my husband has grown to love my bald head as much as I do.

Not having hair draws attention. There have been many times I was sitting having dinner at a restaurant or out with friends when someone would walk up to me and take my hand and ask if they can say a prayer for me. I can only assume they think I am undergoing cancer treatment. I always let them say a prayer because everyone needs an extra prayer sometimes and I don't ever want to discourage them from praying for others.

I find it funny when someone calls me "sir" before they realize I'm *not* a "sir" and the quick "I'm sorry" that follows. The innocent comments from children are my favorite. Children will often ask, "Shouldn't you have hair?" or "Are you a boy or a girl?" My favorite comment came when my husband and I were in an elevator with a young boy and his father. The young boy had beautiful hair. After looking at me, he turned to his dad and said, "I wish I could give her some of my hair." His father turned bright red with embarrassment as the boy just smiled. I smiled at the boy and turned to the father and said, "Don't be embarrassed, the innocence and honesty of your child is beautiful." In the end, hair is just hair and my not having any makes me happy, makes me feel beautiful, and allows me to offer hope to others.

14

WALKING AWAY

From the time I was first diagnosed, I knew I had a gift. A gift of being able to understand how to help people who were newly diagnosed with cancer cope with the life-changing information. When I found out about a dream job of working with pediatric cancer patients, I immediately applied. To my surprise, five months later I was about to start my next adventure.

I began living my dream. I had always wanted to work with pediatric cancer patients, and now I was. I worked as a recreational therapist/child life specialist, primarily with the hematology/oncology patients. On my first day of work, I felt I was where I was supposed to be; my dreams were now a reality.

In this job, you first must prove you understand various procedures before you can start doing procedural preparation with your patients. My supervisor and I sat down so she could demonstrate how she preps a child who is getting an IV. I was the child; she was the therapist. She went step by step, with an actual butterfly needle (the needle part was broken off for safety reasons) and when she got to the needle prick she said, "You will feel a little prick, but then the nurse pulls the needle out and all that is left is a tube, like a straw, in your vein, and that is how you will get your medicine." I said with disbelief, "Wait, the needle doesn't stay in my hand? It's just a straw?"

During my entire treatment, I thought when I received an IV, the needle part stayed in my hand. I also thought I was an idiot for not realizing the needle was removed. I thought back to the anxiety IVs in my hand or arm gave me because I was terrified to move my arm where the IV was, for fear the needle would also move. So, I always had the nurse tape my arm to a board to keep it immobile.

This experience showed me how much I missed out by not having a recreational therapist or child life specialist. I realized how nice it would have been for someone to have taken the time to explain things to me, show me what was going to happen. Maybe my nurses thought I didn't need the extra explanation because I was a teenager, but I know now you can't assume what patients know. You can't assume they understand. Realizing this made me a better therapist.

I loved my job. I loved being able to help my patients and their families understand their diagnosis in a developmentally appropriate way. My favorite time with the patients was their first hospitalization, when they were newly diagnosed. I loved teaching them about their cancer and the procedures they would be having, being there during those procedures to help them cope, and playing with them so they could feel normal.

There were many parts of my job I loved. I gave sock monkeys to patients. Together we practiced medical procedures and I let the child play doctor with these monkeys. When the child would have surgery to have a central line placed, I did surgery on the monkey, so when the child woke up, the monkey had a central line too. I gave the teenagers a sense of normalcy by playing guitar hero, basketball, or a game of pool. I put calming music in the rooms of dying patients. I gave notebooks to parents so they had a place to write down all their questions and clear their minds of the "what- ifs."

The "what if" notebook, as I call it, is something I recommend to everyone affected by cancer. When you are lying in bed at night, thoughts can just race through your head. The best thing to do is write them down, not only so you can clear your head, but also so you don't forget, and you can ask the health care team about them later.

Each patient was different, but regardless of what we did as part of their therapy, I knew it was making a difference in their lives. One patient hated how the chemotherapy changed his sense of taste, so to make his hospital stay better, we would always cook a steak the day he was admitted. There was a kitchen in the therapy room for staff to use with their patients. His nurses were great and would wait to start his chemo until after his steak dinner.

I had patients who always had their heads covered by a hoodie or blanket. I knew they were listening, so I did everything with their mom or dad so they could hear. I had to meet the children where they were. These children were not ready to face things head-on, but they listened to every word I said.

One day I received a call from the outpatient clinic. One child, who I never worked directly with during his hospitalization because he was always hiding under something, was asking for me specifically to help him through a procedure he was about to have in the outpatient clinic. With a smile on my face, I quickly went to the clinic to help this child. I knew he had been listening to what I said the whole time I had been talking with his parents, and because I respected his need to be a passive observer, I had gained enough of his trust that he wanted me by his side on his first outpatient visit.

For the first year, I thought everything was great. Then I had my one-year review. During my initial interview for the position, my boss stated I would not be able to disclose my own experience of cancer to my patients. At the time I honestly didn't take what she said at the interview into consideration, because I saw being a cancer survivor as something positive. I soon found out my boss didn't see it that way.

During my review, she reiterated she did not want me disclosing the fact I was a survivor to my patients and nursing staff. I was surprised. I had worked there a year and hadn't disclosed anything, so why would she think I would start telling people now? Did she not trust my professionalism? I know many cancer survivors who work in the medical field, specifically hematology and oncology, because they can relate, and their bosses see it as a positive attribute. I've seen firsthand what a difference it makes when talking with someone who has been through it. When I was going through cancer treatment, all my doctors voluntarily had a bone marrow biopsy and spinal tap so they could tell their patients what it felt like. This is something I always admired in my doctors; they didn't have to do it, but they chose to so they could comfort their patients.

There is a huge difference to a child when you say, "I *know* what it can feel like" vs. "I've *heard* what it can feel like." Sadly, I had to talk to my patients from a third-person perspective.

I saw what my mentor did for me, and it was nice having someone who could tell me what to expect. I saw the effect I had on a girl I mentored who also had leukemia. She was a few years younger than I was and lived next door to my uncle. On the day we met, she told me her biggest fear was getting her Broviac out. She was scheduled to have it removed soon and she was terrified. She was afraid that when the catheter was removed, she would be left with a hole in her chest. It had only been a few months since I had mine removed, so I showed her my scar. I showed her how skin grows over the hole, and at that moment, I could see the anxiety leave her. Even though I was able to ease her fear that day by showing her my scar, I also knew I wouldn't be showing my scars to any of my patients.

I believe my boss had boundary issues and was afraid I would cross the line. I wonder if she thought I would just burst into a room and declare, "Hey, new patient that I have never met before, I am a cancer survivor. Let me tell you what to expect." I did not feel she valued the fact I was professionally trained to be a recreational therapist and child life specialist, or that I would use my knowledge of what it was like to be a patient to be more compassionate. My experience gave me a deeper understanding of what it was like to be a patient, especially a teenage patient. I played with my patients as much as I did therapeutic sessions such as procedural preparation and medical play. I saw the value of having sessions that were unrelated to cancer, sessions where they could feel like a normal teenager.

I did talk to my boss about my feelings. I told her about other hospitals that hired survivors and were excited for them to help their patients. The hospital I was working at had a burn unit. I told her I didn't have visible scars as a cancer survivor. I asked if she would hire a recreational therapist for the burn unit who was a burn survivor with visible scars? She couldn't answer the question. She couldn't see the value of having survivors help survivors. My attempts to make her understand always fell on deaf ears.

Even though I hadn't disclosed anything thus far, I soon felt I had to hide a big part of me at work, but I did find ways around it. When a child went on their Make-A-Wish trip to Disney World, I would tell them to say hi to Mayor Clayton Rabbit, something only someone who was a Wish Kid would know. I had a greater understanding of what a child might be going through. At one point a mother couldn't figure out why her son was suddenly putting up a fuss when it was time to take his medicine. He had never done it before, and she couldn't understand why he was acting that way. I suggested it might be because school had started and he wanted to be normal. He wanted to be like the rest of his friends. She agreed and thanked me for my insight.

Another time, I was helping a young girl who was recently diagnosed. Her hair had just begun to fall out and she, like me, enjoyed pulling it out. Her mom, as supportive as she could be, just couldn't understand this. I explained it doesn't hurt when you pull your hair out. This gave the mother some comfort. I wish I could have been able to tell her mother I did the same thing, but I couldn't, I could only offer the third-person advice.

On one occasion, I was helping a patient relax during a procedure. The doctor who knew I was a survivor asked if I had local anesthesia when I was going through treatment. I felt uncomfortable because I was there for the patient and I wasn't supposed to talk about it, but I replied no and explained I only had Emla cream. The nurses in the room were surprised. They had no idea I was a survivor and asked me why I never mentioned it. I simply replied that I wasn't allowed to. They were amazed because they saw the benefits and hope I could share with my patients and families if they knew.

Some of the parents and nurses questioned my insight. Some started putting two and two together and would ask if I had ever had cancer. I was honest and told them yes. When they found out I was, in fact, a childhood cancer survivor, their comments were "Why didn't you tell us?" or "You could have given us so much hope." or "That explains so much and why you understood what my child was going through."

I wasn't ever going to tell a patient unless I knew I could offer hope or words of wisdom. At one point, a patient was scheduled to get his central line removed. His mom, a teacher, was worried that school was starting soon, and he was going to be around a lot of people. She was worried he would get sick and end up back in the hospital and need his central line for antibiotics. This mother was one who put two and two together. She wanted the opinion of a cancer survivor, not of a health care worker. So I gave her the same advice my mentor gave me: keep the central line in for a few more months. See how his body responds to being around people, and if he doesn't get sick, then remove it. She appreciated my honest answer.

Shortly after I shaved my head for the St. Baldrick's Foundation, a colleague was working with a teenage patient who had been in an accident. The accident was going to prevent her hair from growing back. Knowing her patient was never going to have natural hair again, and how much hair means to a teenage girl, my colleague thought it might be a good idea for me to meet the patient.

When I walked in the room, the girl was happy to see a confident, successful bald woman in front of her. This gave her the confidence she needed to look in the mirror for the first time since her accident. We looked in the mirror together and talked about what she saw. I explained you don't have to have hair to feel beautiful; beauty comes from within. I went on to work with the girl to help her cope with the loss of her hair and help her understand hair doesn't define you. I informed her that there are so many great wigs available now and she could have fun changing her hairstyle as often as she liked. She and her family were left with hope. It wasn't the false hope that my boss was worried about, it was true hope.

Keeping my secret hit me the hardest when my parents came to visit. I had hoped my parents would get a chance to see me walk in the survivor lap in The American Cancer Society's Relay for Life event at the local college. I wanted them to feel proud of what I had accomplished, but to my surprise, when I got to the relay and found my name in the program listed under Survivors, Dad immediately said, "What if someone at your job sees this?" I know he was concerned about my job, but he should never have had to feel that way. Pride or joy should have been his first emotion. In my opinion, being a survivor should never have been an issue, but unfortunately, my personal life was being affected by my work life.

I do believe there are people who don't believe a survivor can separate their own experience from those of their patients. But you can. You take your own experience and use that to be more compassionate, to be more under-standing, and at times to offer hope.

Many childhood cancer survivors find careers in health care. Why? Because they want to give back, they want to help in the same way their nurses and doctors helped them. I became a recreational therapist/child life specialist because when I was sick, I didn't have one. Through my classes and clinical training, I realized if I had had a child life specialist, I would have had a greater understanding of what I was going through, and I may not have been such a pain to the nurses. As a professional, you realize everyone's journey with cancer is different, and you can never compare your own to your patients.

In the end, I quit the job I loved because I was tired of living two lives: hiding my cancer at work yet volunteering and advocating for cancer survivors in my personal time. For the first time, I had to take a break from the cancer world. I stopped volunteering for cancer organizations I had been a part of for years. I walked away from everything cancer.

15

VELVET

*K*nowing my cancer history, people always asked me if I would have children. My response was always the same: if it is in God's plans . . . yes. I wasn't going to let the fear of my child having cancer stop me from having children. To be honest, I didn't know if I could even have children. I didn't know if cancer treatment affected my fertility and I was all right with the thought of never having a child of my own. The only thing I did know was that I would have dogs: at least some of my children would have four legs, fur, and a tail. What I didn't know was that my first dog would be diagnosed with cancer and I would finally know what it felt to have someone you love, someone in your family, be diagnosed with cancer.

I always knew I would adopt a dog after I graduated from college. When I was sick, I missed my dog the most. I wanted a therapy dog; one I could train and take to hospitals and nursing homes to make people smile. A few weeks after I graduated from OSU, I decided to head to the local animal shelter to look at dogs. As I walked the dog wards, a thin brown dog caught my eye. I was able to take her out of the cage to get a closer look and fell in love with her. She had the sweetest face and the softest fur, and she only had eyes for me. It didn't matter what was going on around her, she just wanted to be with me. She was a beautiful brindle German Shepherd/Whippet mix. I knew I couldn't take her home. I was living with my parents and I needed to make sure they were going to be all right if I brought a dog home. I put her back in her cage, knowing I would be back to have a second look. A few hours later, when Mom got home from work, I convinced her to come with me to look at the amazing dog I found. On my second meeting with Velvet, I knew she would be coming home with me, so I officially adopted her.

The staff was thrilled she was finally getting a home. Velvet had been in the shelter for two months and was even featured as the dog of the week on the news, but no one had shown interest in her. I believe Velvet was meant to be my dog and I was meant to be her person. I took home one of her flyers and as we walked out the door, I decided to keep the name Velvet since it was so fitting with her soft fur.

Later that year, Velvet and I moved to Toledo to begin graduate school and work on her becoming an official therapy dog. She was a natural. Her desire to be around people and to please me made her an incredible therapy dog.

There were so many people she helped. Jenny at the nursing home never spoke a full sentence let alone words that made sense, but when she saw Velvet, she said, "The brown dog." Then Velvet met Susan. Susan was also a nursing home resident and loved dogs. Due to Susan's disease process, she was nonverbal, and her hands and arms were contracted, which limited her range of motion.

No one knew what she understood anymore because she had lost her ability to communicate. One day when Velvet was visiting, I moved Susan's hand to feel Velvet's fur. I let go to talk with her sisters. Susan moved her arm on her own and grabbed Velvet's tags with her fingertips to look at them intensely. She then took Velvet's leash between her fingers. I stood there talking to Susan and her sisters about Velvet for a half hour, and when it was time for us to go, I asked Susan if I could have Velvet's leash back because we had to go see other residents. Tears began to fall down Susan's face. I looked at her sisters and before you knew it, we were all crying because we knew Susan understood and didn't want Velvet to leave.

Velvet also helped a priest who had a stroke regain the fine motor skills he needed to pick up Communion by picking up her dog food and playing a game of catch with her. Velvet made regular visits to Margaret. She chose not to get out of bed anymore and when Velvet came to visit, she always asked if Velvet could jump in bed with her. Margaret would proceed to tell me about all the Irish Setters she had and the trouble they would cause. Margaret smiled and laughed when Velvet was around and would tell her children about Velvet's visits.

When Margaret passed away and I went to the funeral home to say goodbye, her daughter asked me where Velvet was. It was then I learned that if a dog has played a significant role in someone's life, it is more than all right to take them to the funeral home to say goodbye. I also realized Velvet not only brought joy to Margaret's life but to her family's lives as well, as they knew how happy Velvet made their mother.

During the last four years of Velvet's life, I knew something wasn't right. The lymph nodes in her neck were swollen, yet the initial blood test and biopsy done by her veterinarian came back inconclusive. He suggested I take her to a veterinarian oncologist for more tests. We arrived at the oncologist's and waited to be called to a room. I felt anxious. I didn't know what the doctors were going to do, and I knew Velvet wouldn't understand what was going on. I thought to myself, this is what my parents must have felt like. We finally were called to a room and the vet tech and doctor told me they would take Velvet to the treatment room, where they would give her local anesthesia and do another biopsy, more blood work and take x-rays.

I explained that Velvet didn't like cages; she chewed her way through a metal one when she was younger, and that I would prefer that she not be put in one. They assured me she would be heading right back to the treatment room. I said good-bye to Velvet, told her it would be all right, and I would see her in a little bit. She walked out of the room with the vet tech and I went back to the waiting room. I anxiously sat there waiting to get her back, thinking about how often I sat waiting in the clinic. This time I didn't hear children playing or crying; I heard dogs barking. I saw dogs come out with cones on their heads and people smiling when their beloved pet returned to them.

Eventually, the vet tech came to get me and explained Velvet did great; she was waking up in the back on a soft blanket in the middle of the treatment room. A little while later, Velvet was brought to me, her tail wagging. She was as happy to see me as I was to see her. Dr. Megan told me these tests were also inconclusive, but there was a strong probability Velvet had lymphoma because the symptoms pointed to that.

Yep, you heard it: my dog had cancer. This news was heartbreaking for me, and I took her diagnosis of cancer worse than my own. We made an appointment to come back and she started chemotherapy. It was a once-a-week pill and, sadly, had no effect on her. I kept her on the medication for about two months before I decided the toxicity of the chemotherapy was too great a risk especially since it hadn't done anything for her and was causing her to have trouble controlling her bladder. She frequently had accidents in the house. Her lymph nodes remained swollen and her blood work hadn't changed, so I discontinued the chemo. Due to her health, I retired Velvet from therapy work and let her be a dog.

She lived with swollen lymph nodes. Even though no one could tell me definitively why, I knew something was causing the swollen lymph nodes. Her story mimicked mine: Just like no one could tell me why my back hurt, no one could tell me why her lymph nodes were swollen. No one had answers; no one could tell me what was wrong with her.

Velvet eventually developed a cough, again a sign something was wrong. One day, when her veterinarian was cleaning her teeth, he took an x-ray while she was under anesthesia. In the bottom of the x-ray was her chest cavity and in her chest was a tumor. He officially diagnosed Velvet with cancer. It wasn't lymphoma but thymoma, a tumor in her chest cavity. The tumor was pushing on her heart and lungs, which was causing the coughing and swollen lymph nodes. When he told me she had thymoma, my heart sank, but I was relieved I finally knew what was wrong with her. The difference this time was there was no cure; she was a twelve-year-old dog and surgery was not an option.

I had always been the survivor or friend; I had never been in the role of the parent. I finally knew how my parents must have felt when I was diagnosed. I felt helpless and sad. I wish I had done more with her and I hated seeing her suffer. Her diagnosis of cancer hit me hard. I knew there was nothing I could do to stop the tumor from growing, so I put her on doggie hospice and controlled her pain. I loved her and let her live out the rest of her days with me as happy as she could be. It was hard to see the good in her situation; she didn't have a cure, she was a dog, and she had what I considered a ticking time bomb in her chest.

When she was first diagnosed with probable lymphoma, I decided to retire her from therapy dog work. I didn't want to add more stress to her life than I needed to, but after her official cancer diagnosis, I brought her back to work with me so we could spend more time together. This is when I realized her cancer *did* have a purpose.

Velvet's last therapy visit was with Max, who had terminal cancer and loved dogs. When I told him Velvet was also dying of cancer, he said with a smile, "She's just like me." Her visit made a difference to him. She gave him one last opportunity to pet a dog and relate to someone. Cancer had connected the three of us, and I left work knowing Velvet and I had comforted Max. He died a few days later.

Velvet's cough continued, and I knew it wasn't going to get better. No one could give me answers on how fast her tumor was growing, and I was terrified to see her die in pain. From the time I was told she had thymoma until the day I said goodbye, all I wanted to do was comfort her. I wanted her to know she wasn't alone. I was filled with all the memories we had shared together. Even though she was just a dog, she was *my* dog and my family. Twelve years after I brought her home, I said my final goodbye to the best dog ever and sent her to the Rainbow Bridge.

16

DEATH

$\mathcal{D}$eath is a part of life. You cannot hide from death and it is inevitable someone you know will die. My view of death is different from most. I didn't grow up fearing it. I grew up with the understanding that when someone dies, you celebrate the life they lived, not the one they lost. My grandpa designed monuments for a living, including headstones. Many of my favorite headstones designed by him celebrated the person. Cemeteries and death have never bothered me, probably because driving through cemeteries allowed me to see his work.

In my mind, death means peace. The person who died is whole again and watching over us from Heaven with God. When I was diagnosed, I realized my own mortality. I didn't believe cancer would kill me, but I knew one day I would die. So, when I was fourteen years old, I planned my funeral. I picked the songs I wanted to be played and told my family Katie would be buried with me. I knew I wanted my funeral to be upbeat, not sorrowful. I wanted people to celebrate my life, not cry because I was gone.

I had patients who felt this same way too. One of them

was battling a brain tumor and he knew he wanted the Sixx AM song "Life is Beautiful" played at his funeral. He didn't want people crying because he had died; he wanted people to see the beauty in his life. To this day I can't hear that song without thinking of him.

Death is all too common in the childhood cancer world. And sadly, each year at camp some campers didn't return. Heme Camp had a special tradition to recognize this and honor each camper who didn't come back. Regardless of which campground we were at, one activity remained the same—Rock Painting. This was an activity where campers and counselors would paint a rock in memory of a camper who had passed away. It didn't matter if the camper had only been to camp one year or five years, if they were part of the Heme Camp family and they passed away, a rock was painted for them. The rock was painted with things the camper loved, like their favorite color, sports team, etc. At the end of the activity, we celebrated their lives and honored each child.

"Uncle Dave" Stephens, facilities camp director at Camp Cotubic, was so touched by this activity that he made an official rock garden just for our camp. Each year more rocks were added. The rock garden was a place where staff and campers found healing and closure in celebrating the lives of the children who had passed away.

Then one year everything changed at Heme Camp. There was a new hospital camp director and she felt the rock painting did not belong at camp. Her only explanation was that she felt it was an inappropriate activity. I couldn't have disagreed more. Painting the rocks and placing them in the rock garden was a voluntary activity. Maybe not everyone felt like joining in, but for those counselors and campers who did partake, it was an appropriate and very cathartic way to walk the journey of grief. The rocks were not just rocks. The rock garden provided an opportunity for all of us who knew the children to celebrate their lives by honoring them. One counselor said, "Painting the rocks before the campers arrive at camp brings us back to reality. The reality of knowing this could be our campers' last year motivates us to make this year the best year for the campers who will be arriving." It also gave some campers comfort in knowing if they died, they would have a rock placed at camp and not be forgotten.

Eventually, Heme Camp ended. The hospital didn't see the benefit of the camp and therefore ended it without a real explanation. The end of Heme Camp was the end of an era. I attended for fifteen years, two as a camper and thirteen as a counselor. It was a place where we were reminded of how short life is and how we need to take time from our busy lives to enjoy the little things. The rock garden created at Camp Cotubic is still there. The names have weathered, but the memories remain.

My first experience with knowing someone who died from the same cancer I had was only one year after my diagnosis. My family received a call to pray for Jon, a senior at my high school, because he was in a coma at a local hospital. I didn't personally know Jon, but my family did because he played the drums with my brother in the school marching band. Within a few hours, it was determined his coma was caused by undiagnosed leukemia. Unfortunately, Jon died a few days later. His death allowed me to see what my future could have been. I saw what would have happened to me if my dad had not said enough is enough and taken me to the emergency room. I saw the grief on Jon's parents' faces, and I coped with it the best way I knew how. I believed Jon died because God wanted to start a band and Jon was the best drummer there was. I don't believe God intentionally causes us pain or causes people to die, but I needed to believe there was a reason Jon died and I was still alive.

One month later, my mentor Kelly died. One of my doctors introduced Kelly to me in clinic a year earlier. She was the first person I knew who had been diagnosed with the same kind of cancer I had. She was two years ahead of me in treatment and was able to answer my questions, ease my fears, inspire me, and give me hope. She was the one who convinced me to keep my Broviac for a few months longer than the doctors were recommending. My doctors suggested I have my central line removed prior to starting my freshman year of high school. I was eight months into treatment and had just entered a phase where the need for a central line decreased. The doctors wanted it removed because IV chemotherapy isn't as frequent in the last phase and the risk of infection increases the longer you have a Broviac. Kelly and her mom disagreed with the doctors and suggested I wait a few months. They reasoned that I had not been around a large group of people in almost a year and my immune system was still recovering. There was a high risk of me getting sick and ending up back in the hospital.

I'm glad I waited, because Kelly was right. I did get sick and was hospitalized for three weeks at the beginning of the school year. If I had listened to the doctors, I would have had countless needlesticks to receive the IV antibiotics they were giving me. Instead, they were able to use my central line, making the hospitalization easier and more tolerable.

Sadly, Kelly's leukemia did not respond to chemotherapy and eventually she needed a bone marrow transplant. When her body didn't respond to the transplant, she was my first cancer friend to lose their battle. I was getting dressed for school when my mom got the phone call. It was heartbreaking. First Jon and now Kelly, both from the same kind of cancer I had. I thought to myself, does anyone survive? When Kelly died, she was a freshman in college and was the only person I knew to have survived that long, so I thought I guess I'll be lucky to make it to my freshman year of college. For the first and only time, I was afraid of leukemia, afraid of having cancer. I thought it would kill me too.

My brother and I were never close, but he noticed a change in me. He didn't like the way I was thinking, so he pulled me into our living room, sat me down, and said, "Carolyn, you are not the one who died. Stop feeling sorry for yourself and move on. Yes, it's sad Jon and Kelly died, but you won't. You've come this far, and I know you will beat this." After thinking about what Steven said, I was able to turn my sorrow into gratitude. I was grateful for being alive, grateful for the opportunity to know Jon and Kelly, and grateful for my brother. He wasn't there in the hospital, but he was there for me when I needed someone the most.

Years later, I heard a cancer survivor say, "Cancer is not a death sentence, but rather a life sentence that pushes us to live." I realize now that my brother knew this. He was pushing me to live. I used Jon and Kelly's deaths as motivation to live my life. I wanted to live because they couldn't. I wanted to live so I could share their stories. Everyone's life has a purpose, no matter how long they live on the Earth. Their lives helped me understand what was happening to me. Their deaths helped me understand my future.

A wise person once said there is a reason why you meet people when you do. Some people are in your life for a short time and others are there to stay. Some people are here to teach you a lesson, while others are here for you to teach.

Years later, Amanda taught me about life, death, hope, faith, and what being a survivor meant. Amanda was diagnosed with pancreatic cancer when she was twenty-three years old. We met at a cancer survivor meeting in North Carolina. We sat next to each other at the meeting and when it came time to fill out demographic information, we realized we lived in the same apartment complex and we could see each other's apartment from our balconies. I only knew Amanda for a short time, but people don't need to be in our lives for long for their lives to impact our own. What I loved and admired about Amanda was even though she knew her prognosis wasn't good, she never lost hope, she never stopped fighting, and she was always smiling.

Amanda died in 2009. Her death was another reminder that cancer can give, and cancer can take away. It's easy to stay positive when your prognosis is good, but Amanda stayed positive even when facing her own mortality. She lived with hope and faith every day. Amanda understood that death did not mean losing your fight to cancer. She knew that the way you lived, after being diagnosed, was how you beat cancer. She died knowing she wasn't going to let cancer win. She died on her terms, not cancer's.

Like Amanda, David was another friend who lived with hope while facing his own mortality. He was diagnosed with rhabdomyosarcoma shortly after he was married. I met David at a support group for young adult cancer survivors. Little did I know the fun we would have and the heartbreak I would experience when he was gone.

Death may be a part of life but losing someone never gets easier. I have known and loved many people who have gone before me. But David's death hit me harder than anyone else's and I finally felt survivor's guilt. Why did I survive? Why did he die? These are questions I kept asking myself. But then I remembered all the good times we shared.

David and I were the two oldest members of the young adult cancer survivors' group. Afterward, we continued to talk and somehow we got to the subject of Stupid Cancer, an organization I was volunteering for. Hockey Fights Cancer night with the Carolina Hurricanes was coming up and David knew people associated with the team. He set up a meeting and we were in. We explained what the Stupid Cancer Foundation did. It was an organization for young adults with cancer, and the Hurricanes said we could be a part of their Hockey Fights Cancer night. Prior to the meeting, David and I talked about asking to ride the Zamboni. At the end of the meeting, we played the cancer card. We asked and were told they couldn't promise anything.

Hockey Fights Cancer night arrived. David, his wife, Leilani, and I were at the arena passing out Stupid Cancer brochures when they told David and me to go downstairs to wait for a ride on the Zamboni. We were both extremely excited. As we waited, we were at ice level and I remember a puck coming straight toward us and hitting the glass right at eye level. Pretty cool. As we rode the Zamboni, we waved at the audience and they waved back. I never realized how much ice comes off the rink. When I got off the Zamboni, one of the employees gave me his Hockey Fights Cancer pin. It was a night to remember and I am glad I got to share it with David.

Sadly, David died in 2010, seven years after his diagnosis and after having chemotherapy, radiation, and three amputations due to multiple relapses. I was with him at the hospital for his last amputation and remember the love and laughter of that day. He went into surgery with a positive attitude and hopeful his cancer would be gone. The courage and determination he and his wife had as they continued to fight his cancer and live each day to the fullest was inspiring.

It's one thing to have strength, hope, and faith when you know the chemo is working, but it's another to have it when you relapse and treatment isn't working. For many years, I thought of my cancer as a blessing; it had changed my life in such a positive way. When I was sick, I was a witness to God's greatness. Even though I witnessed the faith David and Amanda had, their deaths were my breaking point. I couldn't help but focus on all the things cancer had taken from me.

After saying goodbye to Amanda and David, I got angry. I was already feeling depressed and I was tired of losing friends, tired of the grieving process, and tired of trying to understand why I survived and they didn't. I hated cancer and for the first time saw cancer as more of a curse than a blessing.

When I was diagnosed with cancer, I believed I would survive. There was a purpose for me here on Earth and it had yet to be fulfilled. However, after their funerals, I struggled with understanding my purpose. At this time in my life, I had been dealing with depression for a few years and felt David and Amanda had so much more to offer the world than me. They provided hope and inspired so many people, whereas I wasn't doing much of anything.

I had survivor's guilt. I had a difficult time understanding why some people survive cancer and others don't. Was their purpose on Earth to be fulfilled through their death? When David died, this quote from the Bible was on his memory card: "This illness does not lead to death. It is for the glory of God, so that the Son of God may be glorified through it" John 11:4 ESV. At the time, I did not understand what the quote meant and could not fathom how in

David's last days he turned to this verse. How can the glory of God be shared through death? It took me years to make sense of it. I now know it's in sharing my story, David's story, and Amanda's story, I give glory to Him. The faith Amanda and David had had given glory to God. I am a witness to God's love and greatness. All the things I perceived as a curse were part of God's plan for me and everything happened for a reason. In the darkest moments, God was with me and I grew stronger because of all my experiences—the good and the bad. Through their deaths, I learned to find hope in the darkest moments, to celebrate their lives and my own because we never know when God will call us home.

How I felt about being a survivor changed. At first and for many years, it was about the joy of beating cancer and about living. As I got older, it became more about merely surviving. Surviving the loneliness, the sadness that my friends were no longer in my life because of cancer. The feeling I was alive, and they weren't. The feeling of being different. Being a survivor felt like a black cloud over me. Occasionally I saw through the cloud and saw a rainbow. Eventually, the black cloud disappeared, and I was proud to be a survivor again. I survive for those who didn't. I survive to help others who are newly diagnosed, and to offer hope and encouragement. I am a survivor not because I fought harder but because I believe God had plans for me. His plans for me are through life, not through death.

What I realize now is it is OK to hate cancer—to yell, scream, and cry over a diagnosis. Cancer is an ugly thing. It doesn't discriminate. It doesn't care if you are young or old, rich or poor, black or white. All cancer wants to do is destroy your body. I didn't hate cancer until twenty years after my diagnosis. I wasn't angry I had cancer, but I was angry at everything cancer took from me, which led to depression. I was angry that I was never going to be normal.

In 2009, on my fifteenth cancerversary, I reached the point in my life that life after cancer was longer than my life before cancer. I realized my normal was life after cancer. I thought about what my life would have been like if I had never been diagnosed. What would I have looked like? What would I be doing? What would I have been interested in? What I didn't realize was there is no set normal. Everyone's normal is different and I eventually embraced the fact that my normal included having leukemia. Cancer helped shape who I had become; it led me down the path that God had planned for me.

17

DEPRESSION

*W*hile undergoing cancer treatment, my schedule was completely off. I would get up around 10:00 or 11:00 a.m. and go to bed around 2:00 a.m. My dad hated this, and my mom tolerated it. No one knew I did this on purpose. Every day was the same: get up, take two or three pills, take more pills at lunch, and even more pills before I went to bed. I hated all those pills. I hated knowing as soon as I got out of bed, the cycle would begin again. Each morning I would wake up around 8:00 a.m., but I would force myself to go back to sleep to avoid the day beginning. There were times my mom would check on me and I would fake being asleep just so she would go downstairs and I could lie in bed longer. I stayed up late for the same reason: I didn't want to go to bed. I would take my last pill around 11:00 p.m. and wanted as much time as possible before I had to take another pill. I knew the later I went to bed, the later I slept in.

This cycle got to me one night. I was sick and tired of taking pills. I hated cancer for making me take ten or more pills every day. I was frustrated and upset. I just wanted to be normal. I wanted to be like everyone else. I wanted to be done with cancer. I told my mom I wanted to go to the garage, turn the car on, and die. In my mind, it was the only way to stop the cycle. My mom saw the emotional and mental pain I was in and made the decision I could skip my evening pills. She wanted me to have one night of normalcy. She knew I needed a break. She knew skipping one dose of medication wasn't going to kill me.

I wasn't ever going to kill myself. At the time I believed it was a cowardly thing to do, but I had been pushed to my breaking point and I broke. Luckily, my mom saw how broken I was. I went to bed without taking my nighttime medications. I was a normal kid for one night and was able to wake up the next day with the strength to start the cycle again.

Darkness and despair reared its ugly head years later. In 2007, my aunt was diagnosed with cancer and died three weeks later. A few weeks later, my brother married a woman I thought was his perfect partner. I was so excited to be getting a second sister. Then, a few of my patients at the hospital died and then Jason died. I was out to lunch with my neighbor Kristen when she got a call from the emergency room; Jason, her boyfriend, was there. She wasn't given much information over the phone. I didn't have a good feeling about the situation, so we went to the ER together.

When we got to the ER, Kristen asked to see Jason. The security guard told her she couldn't see him until she spoke to a chaplain. I knew my gut feeling of coming with Kristen was right, because they only call a chaplain when something horrible happens. We just didn't know what yet. The security guard escorted us to a private waiting room, and while we waited, Kristen began to pace. There wasn't anything I could do but just be with her and pray. The chaplain finally came in and gave Kristen the news: Jason had died in a motorcycle accident. The next few moments are etched in my memory. Kristen fell to the ground, hands over her eyes, crying. I went to her and put my arms around her. The chaplain explained Jason died on impact. He then took us back to a room to see him. He was lying on the table, lifeless, blood on his clothes. It was the first time I had ever seen a dead body. I'd been to funerals and seen people lying in a casket, but this was different. Kristen held on to him, crying. I supported her, prayed for her, and I called her sister and her parents who lived a couple of hours away. Her parents eventually got to the hospital and I left. I went home a changed person. I went home with a deep sadness in my heart.

Add everything together and it created the perfect horrible storm. The emotional roller coaster took its toll on me. For weeks I kept replaying in my head, as if it were a movie, being in the ER with Kristen and seeing Jason lying on the table, and depression set in. What was the point of falling in love when it was so easily taken away? I thought about all the things I had lost in my life. First, all my "normal" friends from high school and college, the loss of Kelly, Jon, and my aunt to cancer, the loss of control, my health, and a normal life. My closest friend at the time had just moved away, my relationship with Sam ended, and now I couldn't get Jason out of my mind.

I felt disconnected from everyone and everything. I felt numb inside. I couldn't feel. I didn't feel happy or sad. I felt nothing. I felt empty. The emptiness scared me. I sat in my walk-in closet thinking "I know why people kill themselves," but then I thought about Velvet. She was my why. She was why I couldn't kill myself. I couldn't leave her.

I called one of my coworkers and she came over with another coworker and they convinced me that I needed to seek professional help. I soon began seeing a therapist. I didn't feel loved; I felt I didn't deserve to be loved. Very few people knew about my depression. When you feel numb, you feel nothing, so it's hard to talk about your emotions.

My parents had no idea how I felt until they came to visit me. We were standing in my kitchen and started talking about finances. My dad found out I didn't have as much as he thought I should have in the bank. He got upset, and I told him the reason I had no money was because I was seeing a therapist because I was starting to understand why people kill themselves and that scared me. My parents were shocked. Living in a different state, they had no idea what I was going through.

I found a job in my hometown and moved back home a couple of months later. I needed to leave my job, my boss, and I needed to get away from cancer, from death, from the memories Maryland had given me. I moved in with my parents to save money, but I didn't eat dinner with them. I barely talked to them. I felt I had disappointed them. All I wanted was for them to see how hard it was for me. Happiness was a struggle. I didn't have energy or a desire to do anything. I cried a lot behind closed doors. I cried myself to sleep for two years. I went to work every morning and came home to sadness.

Then came my Golden Birthday. I love celebrating my birthday and this year was special because I was turning thirty on the 30th. When your age coincides with your birthdate, it's called your Golden Birthday. I told my parents I wanted a party to celebrate. I finally was looking forward to something and I was the happiest I had been in a long time.

Family and friends came. We used Care Bear plates and Pound Puppy napkins, which my mom found in a cabinet from a birthday party when I was little, and the cake decorations were the same ones that topped my cakes growing up. For once, I was happy my mom saved everything. On each table were notecards where I asked guests to write a memory of me.

When the party was over and everyone went home, I gathered the notecards to read what people had written. I noticed neither my brother nor my sister had written one. I asked them why not, and they responded that they couldn't think of one. My sadness quickly came back as I wondered how they could not think of one memory with me. I am their little sister. I can think of a million memories with them. I felt they didn't care about me and I instantly regretted moving home.

I felt disconnected from my family. There were times I would be with them and feel completely isolated. My brother and sister-in-law were throwing a party for my nephew's second birthday. I didn't want to go. I wanted to have the house to myself, but I went for my nephew. I knew I would regret not going more than I would regret going. I spent most of the party away from everyone else sitting in their backyard with their dog. I had no desire to be around people.

I was the saddest after being around a group of people, people who had their friends . . . true friends, people who were loved by a significant other. I didn't feel I had true friends. I did have one but felt he didn't count because he lived so far away. Mom saw my sadness and tried to make me happy. Sometimes she would surprise me with a stuffed animal or a card. I appreciated her gestures but sadly, they didn't do much. What frustrated me was I knew she cared, but I just couldn't feel it.

I learned to rely on myself because I lost faith in the world. Not much made me happy anymore. Velvet made me happy, but I also felt ashamed because I wasn't caring for her needs the way I should be. We didn't go for long walks anymore, mostly because it took too much energy. My nephews made me happy, but I rarely saw them because I didn't have the energy to drive two hours to see them.

I felt lost. My life was at a standstill, I couldn't see my future, and the thoughts of killing myself came back. This time though, I had a plan. I knew what I was going to do, but I fought every day against it. I stopped myself from writing a suicide note, because a note was the first part of the plan, and once I had done the first part, the second part would have been that much easier to do and harder for me to fight off. I had nowhere to go to escape the pain and emptiness I felt inside. On May 11, 2011, I hit rock bottom.

This is an excerpt from my journal:

I think it is important to tell my story. My thoughts about suicide—wow, I've never written *that* word before. My original thoughts were about how much my family would miss me. Velvet would miss me. Turned into wanting to write my note and thinking I would do others a favor by killing myself. That was the scariest moment in my life. The moment I realized I was on the edge and had two options. I am choosing to step back from the ledge.

I spoke with another therapist shortly after this was written. I liked this one much better than my first because I felt she listened to me. I described myself as a functional depressed person. I got up every day, went to work, and did what I needed to do to survive. I lost my appetite. I ate because I needed to, not because I wanted to. I would cry myself to sleep every night, and when I was alone, I was filled with thoughts of killing myself. I knew this wasn't a good place to be, but I didn't know how to get out. I wondered if people could tell I was sad, and if so, why didn't they say anything? Were they afraid it would make me sadder?

In my darkest moments of depression, there were times when I looked at my life and I felt broken. I was a fraud. I survived cancer yet wasn't living life to the fullest. For years, I told people life is short and to cherish the moment, but right now, I couldn't do that. I couldn't cherish any moments. I didn't take care of myself the way I should, and I took things for granted. I had always tried to live life with no regrets, but I did—the constant regret was I was not living life the way I should be.

I struggled not only with the negative thoughts but the thought that everyone called me "strong" and "brave" for surviving cancer. I didn't feel strong or brave; I felt ashamed and weak. I didn't want to disappoint people, so I kept everything in. I didn't tell anyone about my sadness, about the darkness, about the suicidal thoughts. I lost my voice. I lost the ability to connect with people, to share my feelings. I had difficulty having a conversation with someone without becoming emotional. I hated myself for bottling everything up. I wanted to be the Carolyn I was before the depression, the happy-go-lucky me. The one thing I wanted most I was preventing myself from having.

Some might say just force yourself to talk, force yourself to open up, but it is easier said than done. Years later, I continued to struggle with opening up and sharing my feelings, which was incredibly frustrating because before my depression I didn't have a problem with sharing my feelings. One thing I learned is you can't ever get out of the darkness by bottling it up. You must talk to someone: a therapist, a family member, someone you trust. By talking with a therapist and making a conscious effort to think positively, my life changed.

I had to find a happy place in my heart. I learned you can't rely on others to make you happy; you have to find it within yourself. I surrounded myself with happy thoughts and kept a happiness journal, forcing myself to find the good in each day. I had to change the way my brain thought, to retrain it to think positively and to focus on everything God had given me. I had to remind myself that even though I felt alone, I wasn't. I had God, Velvet, and parents who loved and supported me.

If I had to describe what it felt like to be depressed, to be so sad, to feel no hope and no happiness, I would tell someone to go watch the Disney movie *Inside Out*. I fought back tears the entire movie because, for the first time, I realized what was happening inside my brain when I was depressed. All my happiest memories were lost, sadness took over, and I couldn't find joy. My islands of friends, family, camp were gone or just hanging on by a thread. By working with my therapist, listening to Christian Rock, and prayer, I was slowly able to find my happy memories. I was slowly able to pull my way out of the darkness and find the strength to connect with people again.

I reconnected with an old camp friend who was taking salsa lessons at Fred Astaire Dance Studio Columbus Northwest. One night everyone from the studio was going out on the town to dance to a live band. I didn't have anything to do and I was longing for a friend, so I went. I didn't plan on dancing. I didn't know how to salsa and I certainly didn't know any other kind of ballroom dance.

Daniel, the owner of the studio, asked me to dance. I told him I didn't know how, and he replied with a smile, "You don't have to." He took my hand, led me to the dance floor, and taught me the basics. All I needed to know was he was the lead, I was the follow, and he would tell me what to do. I had so much fun and the instructors were cute, so I went back to the studio a couple more times with my friend. Daniel didn't know it at the time, but he had given me the gift of dance that night. By taking his hand and going out on the dance floor, my world was about to become a whole lot brighter.

Each Friday night, the studio had a social dance party anyone could attend. I didn't need to know how to dance, because the instructors coached me along the way. At my first party, I met so many other dancers, but the one person who stood out the most was Pat. Pat didn't know she saved my life that day. Pat welcomed me with open arms into the Fred Astaire family by wanting to get to know me and inviting me to the traditional dinner after the party. Pat helped me feel part of something again. For the first time, I felt included. I felt wanted. I felt emotion.

Royce was another dancer. He was a new student as well, so he knew as much or as little as I did. Since we were both beginners, we danced together a lot because we were at the same level. I got to know him, and I felt he wanted to get to know me. I felt I had a friend again. Years later, he told me that when he first saw me, he felt I needed a friend and he felt sorry for me because he thought I had cancer. In his defense, I did have a shaved head and met him when the studio was doing a fundraiser for cancer. He went on to tell me that he was happy he talked to me that day. His friendship, his willingness to break down the wall I had built around myself, helped save my life.

No one at the studio knew I had depression and thoughts of suicide. I was feeling so alone in the world and going to the studio was a last-ditch effort to find somewhere I belonged. To my surprise, everyone welcomed me, everyone made me feel part of the Fred Astaire family. Ballroom dancing allowed me to feel again. It allowed me to be free from thought and just follow. Many times I would leave the studio after a lesson and cry. These weren't the tears of sadness I was used to, but tears of joy. I found something that made me happy. I was happiest on the dance floor, where I was among friends, and I could forget everything when I was dancing. After years of feeling empty and numb, I finally felt again. The studio was a place to go where I was accepted for who I was, where I could laugh and smile and be surrounded by friends.

One month after I started dancing, I was driving in my car when I heard the song "All This Time" by Britt Nicole. As I listened to the lyrics, I started crying, I immediately pulled to the side of the road and sat there with tears falling down my cheeks. I felt the song had been written for me. The words "I know you saw me, hidin' in my bedroom so alone" hit me the hardest. I had been in my bedroom closet when I felt the pain, sadness, and darkness for the first time. I realized when hearing the lyrics that God was with me and had been with me through all the sadness. I had never been alone. Sitting there on the side of the road, I felt a sense of peace. God had been on the journey with me, just as He had when I was fourteen years old. Her song became my anthem. I listened to her song over and over. With all I had lost, I never truly lost God; I had just forgotten about Him because I couldn't see joy, I couldn't see happiness, I only saw darkness. I may have forgotten about Him, but He never forgot about me.

Just as the perfect storm had brought me into depression, the perfect storm brought me out. Through the combination of feeling connected through ballroom dancing, Britt Nicole's song, and talking with my therapist, I finally found peace. I woke up one morning with peace in my heart and a clear mind. Christmas was coming, and I wanted to give my parents something to show them I was all right. Under the tree was a gift for them, a dove ornament to represent the peace I had finally found.

Just as I learned the purpose of my cancer, I learned I had depression for a reason. I met a high school student many years later who was volunteering where I worked. She was a sophomore at the same high school I had attended. She had chosen to come to the rehab center where I worked at the time to complete service hours she needed for school. One day she shared with me her depression and anxiety. We talked for an hour about her feelings, and I shared with her how I understood because I had had depression and knew what it felt like. I left work with a smile on my face. My depression finally had a purpose, and the purpose was to help this young woman cope and understand hers. I also thanked God for having our lives cross paths. I'm pretty sure He knew what He was doing.

Depression is worse than cancer. Chemo fights cancer. Cancer is physical. Depression is mental. Even though you can find relief through medicine, it doesn't cure depression, and because of this I chose not to take medication. I felt I had enough strength inside me to overcome the depression. I had to retrain my brain into rediscovering happiness and joy. I had to remind myself every day that I was never alone because God was always with me and I had people who cared about me. I found other songs that reminded me of God's love and listened to them constantly. "Before the Morning" by Josh Wilson gave me hope I would find joy. "What Faith Can Do" by Kutless reminded me how important faith can be. My heart and mind found peace because I felt God was with me.

I understand why people want to kill themselves. You fight against the thought for so long, you eventually give in, you write the letter and you end the pain. I may have found peace, but I continue to fight the darkness at times. It is very easy to focus on the negatives when something doesn't go my way, and when this happens, I shut down quickly and isolate myself. When I get in these "funks," I get frustrated and angry with myself, but now I have the tools and strength to get out of them. Sometimes a "funk" lasts a few hours and sometimes a day, but I can pull myself out by knowing what I know now: I am not alone, it is OK to not be OK and sometimes it is best to walk away from a situation so you can focus on the positives. Depression is like quicksand that keeps sucking you back in. If you're lucky, someone throws you a rope before you drown in the sadness, the loneliness, the sense of hopelessness. Like quicksand, sometimes it takes a few attempts to get out, out to see the hope, the happiness, and connections in life. No matter what life throws at you, always remember that life is worth living.

TRUSTING GOD

*Y*ou don't have to be religious to have faith. Faith means having complete trust or confidence in someone or something. During my treatment, I not only had faith in God, but faith in my doctors and nurses, faith in my treatment, and faith in myself that I could get through this. Trusting God and having faith He will be there for me comes naturally to me. I have been reminded time and time again that everything happens for a reason. The experiences we go through, the lessons we learn, and the people we meet all have a purpose. Sometimes it's hard to see their purpose and sometimes it takes years to realize it, but the purpose is there and it's not until we sit back and reflect on our lives that we see it. Maybe we go through something so we can help others, not ourselves. At the time of my diagnosis, I couldn't understand how being diagnosed with cancer had a purpose, but I had to have faith that it did. The key thing to remember is we are working in God's time, not ours. It's not easy waiting for God's response to a prayer or to understand why something happened, but we must believe He knows what He is doing.

Cancer or any life-changing event can either push you away or pull you toward your faith. The "why is this happening to me" can been seen two ways—a negative or a positive. You can see it as God has abandoned you, or God trusts you and is by your side. Bad things happen to good people, and sometimes we are in the wrong place at the wrong time, but that doesn't mean God loves us less. It doesn't mean God wasn't there; it means that we are human.

When we trust God, we trust He has a plan. His plan isn't always a happy, easy plan. Sometimes you have to experience something terrible to appreciate the good that came from it. God doesn't give you cancer, but He does help you get through it. I was a sophomore in high school when I first realized why I had been diagnosed with leukemia and why I went through what I did.

When I heard about Jon being in a coma due to undiagnosed leukemia, I asked my dad to take me to the hospital to talk to Jon. I brought a rosary I had been given and a St. Peregrine medal (the patron saint of cancer). When I got to the hospital, I met Jon's father, who was crying. He kept saying, "I should have seen this coming. Why didn't we know something was wrong?" I introduced myself, told him I was a leukemia survivor, and told him there was nothing he could have done. Leukemia has no standard symptoms. His father looked at me and said, "The doctors have been saying that, but I didn't believe it until now." He gave me a hug and I went into Jon's room. I pinned the medal to his pillow and laid the rosary down. I don't remember what I said to Jon, but I know he heard it.

My cancer did have a purpose; it was so I could help Jon's dad and family. It was so I could explain in a way they could hear it that leukemia has no symptoms and there wasn't anything they could have done. I was able to comfort them because of what I had gone through. This was my first experience of being part of God's plan and seeing how everything happens for a reason, even cancer.

I have let God lead me through life. I haven't always known where He was going to take me, but I do know I have been in the right place at the right time to help the people I needed to help because of Him. I trust God guides me to where I am supposed to be when the time is right. When I got my first job at a nursing home, I knew it wasn't going to be a long-term job. A year later I applied for a recreational therapist position at a children's hospital, and guess what they required? One year of experience, and I had one year *to the day*. When I worked at the hospital, I can't count the number of times I was where I was supposed to be. The number of times I was working the weekend when one of my patients died. I was able to be there not only for them but for their family as well. God was directing my life.

One weekend sticks out. This wasn't my normal weekend to work; I had switched weekends with a coworker. This weekend, as I was checking the census, I noticed a former patient had been admitted. She was the patient who enjoyed pulling out her hair, the one I gave a sock monkey to and we did medical procedures to it. After her initial hospitalization, her family decided to go to a different hospital to receive chemotherapy. I hadn't seen or heard about her for months. I discovered her treatment didn't work, and she was at the end of her life. I found soft, comforting music and a CD player. I quietly walked into her room, set up the music, said hello to her parents, and left.

At her funeral, one of her aunts came up to me and

said, "You were the one who brought the beautiful music into her room, weren't you?" I smiled and said, "Yes." I knew God had been working through me to bring comfort to both her and her family. God also guided me through my work with my dog, Velvet. In those moments I could use Velvet to brighten someone's day; for example, when she met Max or the day Susan wouldn't let go of Velvet's collar because she didn't want her to go. God was there.

I trust God's plan. I trust He walks with me through life and I am where He needs me to be. Don't let the fear of "what-ifs" stop you from living your life. Have faith in Him. One of my favorite sayings is: "We know not what the future holds, but we know who holds the future." Sometimes you need to take a leap of faith and trust God is going to catch you.

My life has been full of ups and downs, but one thing I know is God has always been there for me, even in my saddest moments when I have forgotten Him. The Footprints Poem reminds me of this because no matter what is going on in my life, God is either celebrating with me by walking next to me or carrying me because I didn't have the strength to go on.

When I was first diagnosed, Brian was the second person to come see me. He was a seminarian and had gone to the college behind our house and had befriended my brother and me. Even though I was raised Catholic and understood who God was, Brian helped bring me closer to God and see the role He played in my life. Brian told me God was always going to be there for me and He only gives someone as much as they can handle. I guess God thought I could handle a lot.

Brian also introduced my mom and me to Christian Rock. When my mom and I were up late at night, we would watch Christian Rock videos on TV, and we would listen to it in the car on the way to the hospital. The one thing I learned about this genre of music is that the right song plays when you need to hear it. One song had a big impact on me at the time of my diagnosis: "Testify to Love" by Avalon. This song reminds me of what my mom told me shortly after I was diagnosed, that I was a witness to God's love, and I would live to testify His greatness. We each have a testimony to God; we all have a story to tell. This song and others I heard were a constant reminder of God's love and God's faith in me and my faith in Him. These songs helped me when I was fighting cancer, and it helped me again when I was fighting depression.

I grew closer to God during my cancer treatment. My Catholic upbringing gave me the foundation, but my faith and relationship with God developed in the hospital. I trusted and had faith in God, knowing I would survive. It was easy to talk with Him, to ask for comfort, and to give thanks. When I was diagnosed, my mom encouraged me to focus on the positives, focus on the here and now, and focus on the things I was grateful for. When the days seemed long, she would have me focus on an hour, and if an hour was too long, I focused on the minute. It's easier to get through tough times when you break it down into smaller, manageable segments. I thanked God for those moments of energy, those moments of feeling good, and I asked God for comfort when I felt bad.

I'm a firm believer in "guardian angels." I believe they can be as big or small as you need them to be. When I had an upset stomach and I didn't know why it hurt, I would ask my guardian angel to fly inside me to calm my stomach. Each time I did this, my stomach calmed within ten minutes. My guardian angel was there.

I think sometimes we forget guardian angels are around protecting us. I was lucky to know I had one in the first grade. My parents had a friend over for brunch. When it came time to say goodbye, my mom carried me outside, and while going down the four steps in the garage, she missed the last step and fell. She fell on me while cradling my head to protect it from the concrete garage floor. I didn't have a scratch or a bruise, but my mom had a compound fracture and was rushed to the hospital. She always told me her guardian angel worked with mine to protect me.

I prayed for my doctors, my nurses, and those making the chemotherapy and anti-nausea drugs. Each day I would wake up and offer my day to God, and each night before I went to bed, I would thank Him for the good times I had. I saw other kids at the hospital who were much sicker than I was, so I quickly realized there is always someone worse off. Compared to other kids, my treatment seemed easy. I may have spent more time in the clinic getting blood transfusions than other kids, but at least I wasn't as sick as they were. I didn't get the mouth sores my doctors warned me about, and chemo didn't make me as nauseous as the other kids were. I believe my pain was before my diagnosis, so God spared me pain and discomfort afterward.

Prayer works. Each morning I woke up knowing everyone at my grade school and everyone at my brother's high school was praying for me. I was receiving prayer cards from people around the world. I discovered St. Peregrine was the patron saint of cancer and prayed to him and said countless rosaries with my mom. Each prayer helped me get through that moment in time. I felt comfort in knowing so many people were thinking and praying for me.

Once I got home from my initial hospitalization, I continued to receive Holy Communion every day. My neighbor would come over to pray and bring me the sacrament since I was not able to go to church initially because I couldn't be around large crowds. There was a Catholic seminary behind my house, and I had befriended the guys who played soccer. I didn't have many friends in my neighborhood and the soccer field was directly behind our house, so I found it was easy to talk to them. When they heard I was sick, they arranged for one of the priests to say Mass in our home. The seminarians prayed for me and were even kind enough to come and help me with my homework.

One of my favorite gifts was a shirt from my aunt and uncle that said: "Attitude is Everything." I tried to keep this saying in the forefront of my mind when I was having a bad day. I quickly found out how important attitude was. My attitude remained positive throughout my treatments. By trusting God and believing He was watching over me, I believed I would beat my leukemia and never relapse. I was able to keep my spirits up and my head held high. When I was feeling sick or didn't want to take any more chemo, I would remind myself I just had to get through it, and I would never have to do it again. It was mind over matter. With a positive attitude and believing I was going to survive, I could envision the chemo fighting the cancer cells and winning.

When we have faith in God, we trust there will be a rainbow at the end of every storm. There are two ways of looking at things. You can choose the viewpoint that everything is a miracle, or nothing is. God is everywhere. Some people see Him while others are too busy. I was raised to say a prayer for the people involved in an accident when I heard a siren. If I saw a beautiful sunrise, I thanked God for my eyes. Each morning, I thanked God for being alive. I'm lucky because I have two birthdays: January 30, the day I was born, and January 25, the day I was diagnosed. I was given a second chance at life thanks to God.

I'm not one to read the Bible, but this verse speaks to me: "Don't worry about anything: instead pray about everything. Tell God your needs and don't forget to thank Him for His answers. If you do this you will experience God's peace, which is far more wonderful than the human mind can understand." Philippians 4:6–7 LTB. God wants us to talk to Him. He wants us to trust Him. God wants us to see and feel that He is there for us. He wants us to turn our worries into prayer. Worry puts stress on your already stressed body. Prayer gives us strength and resilience. At a time when we are already weak from cancer, why deprive your body of a source of strength?

My Uncle Mike offered me great advice when I was sick. He told me to think of God as a millionaire who wants you to ask for the million dollars, not just the pennies. My uncle wanted me to know it was all right to ask God for the big stuff, not just the little things. God likes when we trust Him to handle the large obstacles in our life. Let go and let God, as Uncle Mike would always say.

You might ask how do I pray? What do I pray about? It's simple, pray about everything. Faith and our relationship with God is personal. Not everyone I meet has the same faith, believes the same thing, or understands why I believe what I do. That is all right. The key is to start somewhere, start by saying, "Hi, God." Prayer does not need to be a formal prayer, like the rosary or Our Father; prayer can just be a conversation. Tell God how you are feeling, what your hopes and dreams are, what you're worried about. When you are struggling and have no words, tell God to listen to your heart. Ask God for his help and have faith He is listening. If you don't get the answers you want right away, don't give up, keep praying.

I also like the quote, "You may not end up where you thought you'd be, but you will always end up where you're meant to be." I never would have imagined that I would end up being a patient at Children's Hospital, and I didn't think I would ever hear the words "you have cancer," especially as a teenager, but I did. Why? Because God had a plan for me. This may not be the path I would have chosen, but it is the path God chose for me.

My life has been a reflection of God's greatness. Some might say, how is God great? You had cancer. You should be angry at God. I say God *is* great *because* I had cancer. I saw firsthand the power of prayer; I saw miracles happen and lives changed. God wants to celebrate with us, so celebrate today! Celebrate the life you have, your family, your friends, and thank God for all of it.

19

BEING A SURVIVOR

I thought of myself as a survivor from day one.

Years later I realized how important thinking of myself as a survivor was. I was at a cancer survivor conference when the definition of survivor came up: You become a survivor the moment you are diagnosed. While working with cancer patients at a children's hospital, I would tell my patients they were a survivor. They often would reply they hadn't survived anything yet, and I would explain what the true definition was. When I did, I could see a sense of relief and empowerment come over them. Attitude is everything, and believing you are a survivor gives you hope.

Surviving cancer isn't easy. First, you fight for your life and go through treatment—chemotherapy, radiation, surgery. Then you fight to regain your place in the world, figuring out how to be normal again. You need to be a healthy survivor, not just physically healthy, but emotionally and mentally healthy as well. You may be surrounded by people who might not understand what you went through. Or need to tell a future boyfriend/girlfriend about your medical past. Learning how to deal with long-term effects of the treatment, fertility, health insurance, and jobs are all new obstacles cancer survivors have to face.

A childhood cancer survivor's journey is never over. The difference between a childhood cancer survivor and an adult cancer survivor is the amount of years we live with the long-term effects. Survivorship becomes part of our lives. It influences our career choices, relationships, and our overall well-being. When I was first diagnosed, I only saw my cancer as a blessing. Then after all the cancer had taken from me, cancer turned into a curse. Today, however, I believe it is a curse *and* a blessing, not one or the other. I also understand you can't grieve unless you have first loved. Grief doesn't just mean the loss of a loved one. We can grieve the loss of a normal life, due to a life-changing event.

I struggled with surviving cancer—not surviving the leukemia but surviving life after cancer. I struggled to find my place in the world, I struggled to fit in. I knew I would survive, but no one prepared me for when my treatment ended. Taking my last dose of chemotherapy was a scary time for me. Chemo was my safety net; I knew it prevented my cancer from coming back. The day I finished chemo, my safety net was taken away. Without chemotherapy would the leukemia return? I had to trust the chemo and radiation did what they were supposed to do: eliminate all cancer cells. To this day, I hate having back pain, I hate not knowing why I'm feeling a certain way. I don't believe my cancer is back, but I am fully aware I have a higher risk for secondary cancers and other health problems.

Cancer treatment is hard, but it is harder on the body when you are a child, because the body is still growing, still developing. For years, I was always sick with sinus infections and colds. I assumed it was an unfortunate side effect of having leukemia. My body was rebuilding its immune system. Years later in college, I discovered how much the chemotherapy affected my immunities. I needed titers pulled prior to going to clinicals. Titers are tests used to measure the amount of antibodies found in the blood. Every titer I had came back negative. I had lost all my immunities to any vaccines I had been given prior to my diagnosis. I asked my doctors if this was normal, and they said no, especially since I had not had a bone marrow transplant. Unfortunately, for me that meant I had to get all my vaccines again.

I was diagnosed with osteopenia, the precursor to osteoporosis, when I was in my twenties. Most likely this diagnosis was a result of the high doses of steroids I had been given. I am at a higher risk of developing cardiac issues and need EKGs and echos done on a routine basis. Depression is one of the most common psychological long-term effects children with cancer develop. My risk of skin cancer is elevated, and due to the cranial radiation, each year I survive my chances of developing a brain tumor increase. These long-term effects are the cost of surviving cancer. Cancer treatment may have lasted only two and a half years, but the effects of the treatment last a lifetime. It can take years to process what we experienced, and we process different parts of it at different times.

The goal is to not let the costs stop you from living life. Are these potential health risks constantly in the back of my mind? Yes, but I silence them to live. I am conscious of them and am proactive with my doctors to do what I can to catch a new diagnosis in the early stages. Living in fear of what may happen is no way to live. All anxiety and worry do is prevent you from enjoying the moment.

We often forget to see the positive long-term effects of

cancer. I have an amazing relationship with my mom because of it. I don't hold back; I say what I mean and am honest with my friends. I have a strong desire to make a difference in the world, and I don't want future childhood cancer patients to have to go through what I did. I have a high pain tolerance and lack a lot of hair on my arms and legs, making shaving so much easier. Most importantly, I try to live my best life, because I know how quickly life can change.

Survivors often feel as if they have been put on a pedestal—if you can survive cancer, you can survive anything. I do feel I can survive anything, but when the slightest thing happens, people are so quick to say, you've been through worse. I agree I've been to hell and back, but it's OK to feel weak, to feel helpless. You can't appreciate the happy times if you are always happy. You have to experience sadness to appreciate that happiness. You have to see the moon to appreciate the sun.

My zoology background showed me how I can compare cancer to nature. Mother Nature and cancer can be relentless, brutal, and devastating, but they can also be beautiful, peaceful, and resilient.

Cancer kills and destroys everything in its path, just like a wildfire, but life comes back after a wildfire, as it does for cancer survivors. Certain plants can only grow after a fire. The Jack Pine and Giant Redwood are two examples. Their thick, hard cones are glued shut with a strong resin. It is only the heat of a fire that can open the cones to release the seeds. The cones and seeds can remain dormant for years, waiting for a fire. We often view wildfires as horrible events, but to these trees, it means growth, it means life.

Greek mythology also talks about life after death. The phoenix was born from the ashes of its predecessor. Just as cancer can kill one life, it can also create a new one. I have met many people who, due to their own diagnosis or after the death of a child, changed careers to something more meaningful, something they felt had more purpose. The thing to remember is there *is* life after cancer.

When cancer touches your life, it changes you, whether you were the one diagnosed, the sibling, parent, or friend. You will never be the same person when it's over. People say I must have been so strong to have survived cancer, but I was strong because I had to be. Granted, I have a strong personality to begin with, but I was strong because I had no choice, I was strong because I trusted God, and I was strong because I was surrounded by doctors, nurses, and people who supported me.

When you are diagnosed with cancer you have two choices—fight cancer or let cancer win. In college I wrote Poem 3 for anyone going through cancer treatment. It was written to give other cancer patients the strength to keep fighting.

Poem 3

The pain and the hurt,
The comfort and the hope.
The life we lost,
Or the one we gained.
The struggle we fight —
Can be won or lost.
Which would you want?
I chose to win and I won.
I chose to live with the pride
I survived.
My pain and hurt turned into prayers.
The comfort and hope turned into dreams.

Being a survivor means each time I hear about someone I know being diagnosed with cancer, my heart breaks because I don't want to see anyone go through cancer treatment. Their diagnosis reminds me of how I can offer them hope and encouragement. It reminds me of my own mortality and that tomorrow is not guaranteed. To be honest, it gets harder the older I get because I see people my age being diagnosed with cancer. Having cancer as an adult is harder than as a child. Children are innocent and don't deserve cancer either, but they don't have bills to pay, children to comfort, and jobs to maintain. Adults have many more responsibilities to deal with. Kids get wish trips and many experiences not offered to adults.

Being a survivor means awareness. Awareness that life is short, that cancer is the number one killer of children. Awareness that we need to find a cause, not just a cure. Awareness that we need to pray for the researchers as much as we pray for the patients, and awareness that everyone's battle is going to be different. I will always be grateful to two individuals who brought this awareness to the forefront and changed the way survivors live. Lance Armstrong, founder of the Livestrong organization, gave survivors a voice. Matthew Zachery, founder of Stupid Cancer, teaches young adults the art of surviving. It's not about finishing chemotherapy; it's about living every day as a survivor. Surviving cancer treatment is only phase one of being a survivor. Surviving as a survivor is phase two. No one prepares you for phase two. One of the motivators in writing my story is to help others with phase two.

I will never forget the day I was at a Livestrong Summit in Columbus, Ohio, when I ran into Matthew Zachary. I had heard about him briefly and knew he had founded an organization for survivors. I had seen his picture, so when I saw him at the summit, I ran up to him like a little girl and stupidly said, "Oh my gosh, you're Matthew Zachary!" He smiled, and that is how I got involved with his organization, Stupid Cancer.

Fourteen years after my diagnosis, there were finally organizations out there for people like me: young adult cancer survivors. Organizations helping people navigate life after treatment. Helping people cope with being a survivor and fitting into the world again. This meant so much because I knew the struggles I had been through and the mistakes I had made. Livestrong and Stupid Cancer meant future survivors had somewhere to go and someone to help guide them.

There are now many organizations connecting cancer patients and helping survivors and their families learn to live again. Everyone's cancer experience is different, but no one has to go through this alone.

20

LIVE LIFE, LOVE LIFE, CHERISH EVERY MOMENT

One thing cancer can do is change our timelines. The goal is to adapt and accept that everything will happen when it's meant to happen. Every milestone I hit, be it turning sixteen, graduating high school, college, or grad school, was always so exciting for me. I picture the teenager sitting in a clinic, just thankful to be alive. I think about all my friends who didn't make it.

The hardest milestone for me to reach was getting married. Over the years I had always pictured myself being married by the time I was 30. Well, 30 came and went and I was still alone. I have struggled with relationships my whole life. I've often been told I don't give people a good first impression. So to meet the right guy was a challenge. I had only had two boyfriends and I had no idea how to be in a relationship. I had become comfortable with being single and the independence it gave me. Deep down I was terrified my cancer, even though it was in the past, would scare someone off. Then I met Lee.

Lee came into my life months after I found peace with my depression. He didn't care I had a shaved head, he didn't care I had cancer, he liked me for me. He accepted me for who I was, flaws and all. I always knew that whomever I was going to marry was going to be worth the wait, and Lee was worth it. Some people asked me how I could marry Lee since he wasn't Catholic and I was. My answer was always simple, if God didn't mean for him to be in my life, God wouldn't have placed him in it. Don't ever let cancer or any other major life crisis stop you from going after your goals. Trust God's timing.

Our lives don't always follow the paths we envision. Sometimes we take detours before we find ourselves on the right path. One thing is for certain, we are always where we are meant to be. Sometimes those detours lead us down paths we never saw coming, new and exciting paths we would never have found on our own.

Shortly after getting married, Lee and I built a house. It was the perfect house, close to my work, lots of room for the dogs to play, and a nice neighborhood. After two years, our lives took a detour. We were forced to sell our house because the HOA didn't like that we had an Akita. So instead of getting rid of our dog, which the HOA wanted us to do, we sold the house and got rid of the HOA. It was at this time we made the life-changing decision to buy an RV, live in it full-time, and travel the country.

Never in my wildest dreams did I ever picture myself living in less than 450 square feet. But here I am, not only living in a small space but loving it. I not only get to see the beauty of our country, but I get to make amazing friends along the way. The lifelong friends I craved my whole life I now have, because of the detour we had to take.

In the end, life is what you make of it. If you look for the positive, you will see the positive, and if you look for the negative, you will find the negative. When I was first diagnosed my nurses, would call me Pollyanna, because regardless of the situation, I was always able to find something positive about it. During my years of depression, I lost sight of the positive things and only saw the negativity in the world. I can tell you, life is more fun when you see the joy in it. The important thing to remember is that bad days will be there, but trust that good days will follow. Life is better when you have faith and hope for the future.

The key to suriving cancer or any life-changing event is to stay positive, have faith, and never lose hope in a better tomorrow.

Even though Amanda died of pancreatic cancer, she knew how to live as a survivor. This is part of a speech Amanda gave at a Relay for Life event. I have kept it as a reminder of her strength. Amanda is an inspiration to all cancer survivors.

At the time of my diagnosis, I was a normal, run-of-the-mill 23-year-old getting settled into a new career and into graduate school. I was just getting used to this new independent life that I had begun to create for myself when my world was turned upside down. I had pancreatic cancer. If you know anything about pancreatic cancer, then you know it's a rare cancer with devastating survival rates. I had a solid pseudopapillary tumor, documented case number 305 in the world.

After a routine CT scan, the doctors informed me that the cancer was back. This time it was in my stomach and there were too many tumors to count. Exactly one year from my diagnosis, my surgeon went in to remove the tumors. After two hours in the operating room, he came out and told my family that much to his astonishment, he couldn't find any tumors. They were all gone! He had no medical explanation for this occurrence. He did say that he wished his other patients had half of the prayers and support that I have, then he would be saving a lot more lives.

My family and I are convinced that this was nothing short of a miracle. Months later, I was told that I had twenty new tumors, ten on my lungs and ten in my liver. I am undergoing chemo again. It's a battle but my past experiences have taught me that surviving this is going to require me waking up and falling in love with the world and life all over again each day . . . no matter how hard the day before might be.

As a fellow cancer patient/survivor I offer you these lessons that I embrace each day: Live "RIGHT NOW." Don't live in fear of the future. How many times have you caught yourself saying "What if such and such . . .?" "What if the cancer spreads?" "What if the treatments don't work?" "What if the chemo causes my hair to fall out?" Filling your mind with "What-ifs" is only going to prevent you from enjoying the moment you have been given. Don't be consumed with what may happen in the future. I'll be the first to admit that it is hard, but you'll eventually appreciate the fact that even with cancer, YOU HAVE LIFE, HERE and NOW.

Even better, don't just live but LIVE RIGHT NOW WITH HOPE. Live in the moment and know that God is going to take care of you. ALL of life, not just parts of it, is in good hands and live with a promise in your heart that even though the future is uncertain and scary at times that everything is happening for a reason. Live with the confidence that you are being guided every step of the way. Not all of these steps are going to be happy and cheerful, some may be filled with pain and sadness. But choose to LIVE with HOPE knowing that He is always there and will take care of you.

And finally, take on the ATTITUDE of a SURVIVOR. A friend shared a quote with me last night. She said, "Anyone can give up, it's the easiest thing in the world to do. But to hold it together when everyone else would understand if you fell apart, that's true strength." I think the most satisfying compliment anyone could give you is for them to tell you how strong you are. And it's all about attitude. It takes a lot to be strong through the terrifying diagnosis, countless decisions, and harsh treatments that are involved with cancer, but if you have the right attitude you can take on the world. Don't view cancer as a death sentence, view it as a challenge and face the battle head-on. A true survivor realizes that cancer may mean death, but MORE IMPORTANTLY, it may mean life. Invest your time in living each day to the fullest, not just waiting for it to pass.

The past three and some odd years of battling cancer helped me discover the wonder of appreciating just how precious life is. There were times that I feared I would never experience peace, feel joy, or believe that life is good. However, I am experiencing that peace; I am feeling the joy of God's love and His gift of love from others. As a result of this ongoing battle, I say "I love you" more. I have found beauty in places that I might not have ever noticed before. But most importantly, I have discovered how important the unconditional love and support from family, friends, and God are. All three of these play a vital role in your support system. I have been blessed with so many angels in my life since I've been sick. People that have helped me face each day with a smile, knowing that in the end, I was going to be just fine.

I'll end with this note: Cancer is definitely not a life path that we choose for ourselves, but it is one that can enrich your life, and those around you, beyond measure.

Do not just survive this experience but thrive as a result of it. Make the most of what you're dealt, give others hope through your survival, and LIVE. Live with hope and a new love for life.

Like Amanda's speech, a Peanuts cartoon said, "We only live once, Snoopy" . . . "Wrong! We only die once. We live every day." We need to stop and appreciate the small stuff. The beauty of a single snowflake, the colors of the butterfly that lands next to you, the softness of our pet's fur, and the fact we are alive—breathing, with blood flowing through our veins. Cancer taught me life has purpose. Our purpose is to find our gifts and use them to make the world a better place.

Many times throughout my journey people have asked, if I could go back in time and change my life, take away the leukemia, the depression, would I? My response has always been the same: I wouldn't! I would do it all over again because I love where the journey has taken me. I don't keep a bucket list of things I am waiting to do when I retire. I cross things off my bucket list as I add them. I don't want to wait to do something, because tomorrow is not guaranteed.

Would I do it all over again? Definitely. Why? Because God's not done with me yet.

ABOUT THE AUTHOR

Carolyn Koncal Breinich is originally from Columbus, Ohio. She currently lives in a motorhome with her husband, Lee and two dogs, Akiro and Scarlet. They enjoy traveling the United States, seeing the beauty it has to offer. She has a strong faith and believes this book is part of God's plan. She wants to change the world for other childhood cancer survivors, so they don't have to go through what she did.

If you are interested in being added to Carolyn's Cancerversary email listing, sign up at:
www.leukemiagirl.com

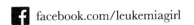 facebook.com/leukemiagirl

Made in the USA
Middletown, DE
12 June 2021

41906988R00106